Dermatosurgery

J. Petres · M. Hundeiker

Dermatosurgery

With a Foreword by K. W. Kalkoff

includes 112 illustrations

Springer-Verlag
New York · Heidelberg · Berlin

Johannes Petres, M.D.
Department of Dermatology
University of Freiburg
Hauptstrasse 7
7800 Freiburg
Federal Republic of Germany

Max Hundeiker, M.D.
Center for Dermatology, Andrology,
  and Venerology
University of Giessen
Giessen, Federal Republic of Germany

Library of Congress Cataloging in Publication Data

Petres, J   1934–
  Dermatosurgery.

  Translation of Korrektive Dermatologie.
  Bibliography: p.
  Includes index.
  1. Skin—Surgery. 2. Skin-grafting.
3. Surgery, Plastic. I. Hundeiker, M., 1937–
joint author. II. Title.
RD520.P4713   617'.477   78-2326

9 8 7 6 5 4 3 2 1

ISBN 978-1-4615-6813-1   ISBN 978-1-4615-6811-7 (eBook)
DOI 10.1007/978-1-4615-6811-7

Dedicated to

W. Schmidt, M.D.
Emeritus Professor of Dermatology,
Medical School of Mannheim, University of Heidelberg,
Federal Republic of Germany

K. W. Kalkoff, M.D.
Professor of Dermatology, University of Freiburg,
Federal Republic of Germany

L. Illig, M.D.
Professor of Dermatology, University of Giessen,
Federal Republic of Germany

Foreword

Dermatosurgery cannot readily be assigned to any one branch of medical science, and as with any borderline case, this assignation is a matter of controversy. Since the end of the last century, the place of the subject in the field of dermatology has been firmly established. This is hardly surprising, since a number of specialists in dermatology spent the first part of their professional life as surgeons: for example, E. Lang of Vienna, famous for his treatment of lupus by plastic surgery; and K. Linser of Tübingen, one of the originators of varicose-vein stripping. H. T. Schreus and C. Moncorps were distinguished members of a later generation of surgery-oriented dermatologists; the dermatosurgery taught and performed in their clinics was of a high technical standard.

The best dermatologist is one who is competent in conservative, radiologic, and operative methods and is thus not dependent on one particular method. The aim of dermatologic training should therefore be to impart the knowledge that gives the dermatologist this freedom of choice. This involves the teaching not only of the basic principles of dermatosurgery but also of the ability to discriminate according to the most varied criteria. In this field, technical knowledge, motivation, and enthusiasm are not enough; talent is also required.

C. Moncorps was engaged in work on a monograph on dermatosurgery (unfortunately nowhere near completion) at the time of his death. As a former pupil and long-standing colleague of his, it is particularly gratifying to me to see colleagues past and present continuing a tradition in their work.

This monograph offers those interested in dermatosurgery material for discussion and for broadening the scope of their knowledge. I wish it a successful reception both within our specialized field and outside it.

K. W. Kalkoff

Preface

Although there are numerous publications in the field of plastic surgery, an introduction to dermatologic surgical therapy still seems needed. A thorough knowledge of skin diseases is required for the successful planning and execution of dermatotherapy, and there are special dermatologic techniques which are not practiced in other specialities. *Dermatosurgery* bridges this gap between dermatology and surgery.

Discussions of the most frequently encountered skin diseases, as well as those which present unusual problems in therapy, begin this book. They include synonyms, descriptions of clinical characteristics and etiology, considerations for differential diagnosis, and possible therapeutic measures. The second section explains the basics of dermatosurgical techniques. This is followed by a survey of the surgical techniques most appropriate to the different regions of the body. The final section is a group of 32 plates of photographs, most showing the preoperation condition, the dermatosurgical technique employed, and postoperative results. A list of over 500 references to the literature, updated for this English edition, provides guidance for readers interested in delving deeper into the subject.

Dermatosurgery does not attempt to replace the specialized literature.

Rather this introduction to and synthesis of the basic knowledge of the subject provides an easy access to available information and increases awareness of therapeutic possibilities. In order to keep the size appropriate to an introduction, we include neither all methods of dermatosurgery nor all technical details. However, the information here will provide valuable insight into the diagnosis and treatment of most problems encountered in clinical practice. Maximum therapeutic results, of course, are achieved by close cooperation with other disciplines.

Freiburg, Giessen, F.R.G.   J. Petres
April, 1978   M. Hundeiker

Acknowledgments

We wish to extend our graditude to Mrs. Waldtraut Petres for her invaluable efforts on the English translation. Mrs. Lilo Goerke and Mr. Thomas Kaut deserve credit for the very fine photography and Mr. Ted Bollmann for the excellent line drawings prepared especially for the English edition. We are also very grateful to the staff of Springer-Verlag for the excellent English text.

Contents

Introduction 1

1. Surgical Indications in Dermatology 3

1.001 Tumors, Preblastomatoses, Cysts, and Malformations 3

1.002 Benign Epithelial Tumors 3

1.003 Basal Cell Papilloma. Verruca Seborrheica 3 / 1.004 Verruca Vulgaris 4 / 1.005 Condyloma Acuminatum 5 / 1.006 Molluscum Contagiosum 5 / 1.007 Verrucous Epidermal Nevus and Rare Epidermal Nevi 5 / 1.008 Nevus Sebaceous (Jadassohn) 5 / 1.009 Clear Cell Acanthoma (Degos) 5 / 1.010 Rare Benign Tumors of the Skin Glands 6 / 1.011 Sebaceous Gland Adenoma 6 / 1.012 Senile Sebaceous Gland Hyperplasia 6 / 1.013 Rhinophyma 6 / 1.014 Nevus Comedonicus 6 / 1.015 Trichofolliculoma 6 / 1.016 Malherbe's Epithelioma 6

1.017 Cysts 6

1.018 Follicle Retention Cysts 7 / 1.019 Traumatic Epidermal Cysts 7 / 1.020 Milia 7

1.021 Precanceroses 7

1.022 Keratoma Solare 7 / 1.023 "Cornu Cutaneum." Compare Molluscum Contagiosum (Sect. 1.006) 8 / 1.024 Tar and Oil Keratoses 8 / 1.025 Arsenic Keratosis 8 / 1.026 Bowen's Disease 8 / 1.027 Erythroplasia of Queyrat 9 / 1.028 Leukoplakia 9 / 1.029 Cheilitis Abrasiva Precancerosa (Manganotti) 9 / 1.030 Radiodermatitis, Roentgenism 9 / 1.031 Lichen Sclerosus et Atrophicans 9 / 1.032 Intraepidermal Epithelioma (Borst-Jadossohn) 10

1.033 Carcinomas 10

1.034 Squamous Cell Carcinoma 10 / 1.035 Carcinomas of the Skin Appendages 10 / 1.036 Paget Carcinoma 10 / 1.037 Skin Metastases of Internal Carcinomas 11

1.038 Pseudocancerous Lesions 11

1.039 Keratoacanthoma 11 / 1.040 Papillomatosis Cutis Carcinoides Gottron 11 / 1.041 Pseudocarcinomous Hyperplasia 11 / 1.042 Oral Florid Papillomatosis 11

1.043 Basal Cell Carcinoma and Related Tumors 12

1.044 Basal Cell Carcinoma 12 / 1.045 Premalignant Fibroepithelial Tumor (Pinkus) 13 / 1.046 Spiegler's Tumor 13 / 1.047 Epithelioma Adenoids Cysticum (Brooke) 13 / 1.048 Nevoid Basal Cell Carcinomas 13 / 1.049 Basal Cell Nevus Syndrome (Fifth Phacomatosis) 13

1.050 Benign Tumors of the Pigment-Producing Cells 14

1.051 Lentigo 14 / 1.052 Lentigo Senilis 14 / 1.053 Nevus Pigmentosus 14 / 1.054 Juvenile Melanoma (Spitz) 15 / 1.055 Nevus Coeruleus 15 / 1.056 Nevus Pilosus 15 / 1.057 Melanophacomatosis (Virchow-Rokitansky-Touraine) 15

1.058 Premalignant and Malignant Neogenesis of the Pigment-Producing Cells (Steigleder and Clark et al. [54, 466]) 15

1.059 Lentigo Maligna, Premalignant Melanosis Dubreuilh 15 / 1.060 Lentigo Maligna Melanoma, Dubreuilh Melanoma 16 / 1.061 Superficial Spreading Melanoma 16 / 1.062 Nodular Malignant Melanoma 16

1.063 Benign Tumors and Pseudotumors of the Connective Tissues 17

1.064 Histiocytoma, Dermatofibroma 17 / 1.065 Nevoxanthoendothelioma 18 / 1.066 Xanthelasmas 18 / 1.067 Xantomas 18 / 1.068 Keloid 18 / 1.069 Hypertrophic Scars 19 / 1.070 Pseudosarcomatous Fasciitis 19 / 1.071 Desmoid Tumor 19 / 1.072 Nontumorous Fibroplasia (see Sect. 1.117) 19 / 1.073 Adenoma Sebaceum in Conjunction with Phacomatosis (Bourneville-Pringle) 19

1.074 Semimalignant and Malignant Tumors of the Connective Tissue 19

1.075 Dermatofibrosarcoma Protuberans 19 / 1.076 Fibrosarcoma 19 / 1.077 Other Sarcomatous Forms 20

1.078 Tumors of the Fatty Tissue 20

1.079 Lipoma 20 / 1.080 Lipomatosis Dolorosa 20

1.081 Benign Lymphoplasias of the Skin 20

1.082 Lymphocytoma Cutis 20

1.083 Malignant Lymphomas and Hemoblastoses 20

1.084 Benign Tumors of the Vascular and Smooth Muscle Systems 20

1.085 Eruptive Angioma 20 / 1.086 Angioma Senile 21 / 1.087 Nevus Araneus 21 / 1.088 Angiokeratoma. (Preferable [231]: thrombosed angioma) 21 / 1.089 Angiokeratoma Akroasphyticum Mibelli 21 / 1.090 Angiokeratoma Inpunctiforme Scroti s. Vulvae Fordyce 21 / 1.091 Fabry's Disease 21 / 1.092 Capillary Hemangioma 21 / 1.093 Cavernous Hemangioma 22 / 1.094 Glomus Tumor 22 / 1.095 Multiple Familial Glomus Tumors 22 / 1.096 Leiomyoma, Angioleiomyoma 22 / 1.097 Granular Cell Myoblastoma 22 / 1.098 Lymphangiomas 22

1.099 Vascular Nevi 23

1.100 Nevus Teleangiectaticus Lateralis 23 / 1.101 Nevus Flammeus Medialis Unna 23

1.102 Semimalignant and Malignant Vascular Tumors 23

1.103 Hemangiopericytoma 23 / 1.104 Hemangioendothelioma 23 / 1.105 Kaposi's Sarcoma 23 / 1.106 Hemangiosarcoma 23

1.107   Tumors of the Nerves and Nerve Sheaths   24

1.108   Neurilemmona, Neurofibroma   24 / 1.109   Recklinghausen's Neurofibrosis   24 /
1.110   Neurofibrosarcoma   24

1.111   Dysplasias, Hyperplasias, and Fibroses   24

1.112   Tylositas Articuli   24 / 1.113   Palmoplantar Fibrosis (Dupuytren's Contracture)   24 /
 1.114   Juvenile Palmoplantar Fibrosis   24 / 1.115   Induratio Penis Plastica   24 /
1.116   Pseudoxanthoma Elasticum   24 / 1.117   Cutis Laxa and Cutis Hyperelastica   24

1.118   Inflammatory and Functional Skin Lesions   25

1.119   Inflammations Originating from Hair Follicles and Sebaceous Glands   25

1.120   Deep Necrotizing Perifolliculitis   25 / 1.121   Dissecting Cellulitis of the Scalp,
Periofolliculitis Capitis Abscedens et Suffodiens   25 / 1.122   Dermatitis Perianalis
Fistulosa   25 / 1.123   Pyodermia Fistulans Sinifica   25 / 1.124   Acne Conglobata, Acne
Abscedens   25

1.125   Inflammations Originating in the Sweat Glands, the Odoriferous Glands, and the Mucous Membranes   26

1.126   Hidradenitis Suppurativa   26 / 1.127   Bartholinitis   26

1.128   Chronic Inflammations Originating around the Vessels   26

1.129   Tuberculosis Cutis Luposa   26 / 1.130   Sarcoidosis (Besnier-Boeck-Schaumann)
27 / 1.131   Cheilitis Granulomatosa (see Sect. 3.044)   27 / 1.132   Deep Mycoses and
Diseases Due to Actinomyces   27 / 1.133   Leishmaniasis   27

1.134   Inflammations that Spread to the Skin   27

1.135   Dental Skin Fistulas   27 / 1.136   Tuberculosis Cutis Colliquativa   27

1.137   Cicatricial Post-inflammatory States and Post-thrombotic Syndrome   27

1.138   Phimosis   27 / 1.139   Superficial Thrombophlebitis   28 / 1.140   Varicosis in
Chronic Venous Insufficiency   28 / 1.141   Small Varicose Dilations of Cutaneous Veins   28
 / 1.142   Pachydermia Vegetans and Papillomatosis Cutis   29 / 1.143   Dermatopathy of the
Leg   29 / 1.144   Elephantiasis Nostras   29 / 1.145   Leg Ulcer   29 /
1.146   Arteriosclerotic and Diabetic Gangrene of the Leg   30

1.147   Lesions Due to Foreign Bodies and Trauma   30

1.148   Foreign Body Granuloma   30 / 1.149   Tattoos and Other Corial Foreign Body
Intrusions   30 / 1.150   Keloid (cf. Sect. 1.068)   30 / 1.151   Traumatic Epithelial Cysts (cf.
Sect. 1.019)   30 / 1.152   Chondrodermatitis Nodularis Chronica Helicis Winkler   30 /
1.153   Callosities, Tyloma   30 / 1.154   Burns and Scalding   30 / 1.155   Chemical Burns
31 / 1.156   Wounds   31 / 1.157   Suture Dehiscence   31

1.158   Functional and Cosmetic Disorders   31

1.159   Axillary Hyperhidrosis   31 / 1.160   Cosmetic Surgery   32

1.161   Lesions of the Nails   32

1.162   Onychomycoses   32 / 1.163   Ingrown Toenail   32

2. Basic Principles of Dermatosurgery: Survey of Surgical Techniques   33

2.001   Requirements and Considerations   33

2.002   Surgical Instruments   34

2.003   Pre- and Postoperative Care   35

2.004   Anesthesia Procedures   38
2.005   Local Anesthesia (for techniques, cf. [11, 330])   39 / 2.006   Local Anesthetics   39 / 2.007   Marginal Wall Anesthesia   39 / 2.008   Conduction Anesthesia   39 / 2.009   Special Regional Anesthesia Procedures   40 / 2.010   General Anesthesia   40

2.011   Incisions and Suture Techniques   41
2.012   Interrupted Sutures   41 / 2.013   Mattress Sutures   41 / 2.014   Continuous Intradermic Suture   41 / 2.015   Removal of Sutures   42

2.016   Surgical Techniques   42
2.017   Skin Biopsy   42 / 2.018   Elliptical Excision with Primary Wound Closure   42 / 2.019   "Dehnungsplastik" (Friederich [19])   43

2.020   Regional Flaps   44
2.021   Z-Flap Technique   4 / 2.022   VY-Flap Technique   44 / 2.023   Advancement Flap Technique   44 / 2.024   Rotation Flap Technique   45 / 2.025   Transposition Flap Technique   45 / 2.026   Island Flap Technique   45 / 2.027   Combination of Techniques   46

2.028   Flaps and Grafts from Other Body Areas   46
2.029   Free Skin Grafts   46 / 2.030   Tubed Pedicled Flaps   47

2.031   Dermabrasion   47

2.032   Electrosurgery   48
2.033   Electrotomy   48 / 2.034   Coagulation   48 / 2.035   Desiccation   48 / 2.036   Fulguration   48 / 2.037   Curettage   49

2.038   Chemosurgery   49

3. Special Techniques for Different Regions of the Body   51

3.001   Scalp   51

3.002   Rotation Flap Technique   51
3.003   Double Rotation Flap Technique   51 / 3.004   Rotation Flap Technique Combined with Free Skin Graft   51 / 3.005   Full-Thickness Skin Graft   52 / 3.006   Transplantation of Multiple Punch Biopsies   52 / 3.007   Surgery for Relaxation of the Scalp   52

3.008   Temporal Region   53

3.009   Caudal Advancement Flap Technique   53 / 3.010   Advancement Flap Technique— Free Skin Grafting Combination   54 / 3.011   Dorsal Rotation Flap Technique   54 / 3.012   Caudal Rotation Flap Technique   54 / 3.013   Free Skin Grafting Technique (Split-thickness Skin Grafts)   55

3.014   Forehead   55

3.015   Rotation Flap Technique   55 / 3.016   Advancement Flap Technique from Both Temporal Areas   55 / 3.017   Double Rotation Flap   56

3.018   Nose   56

3.019   Transposition Flap Technique   57 / 3.020   Double Transposition Flap Technique   58 / 3.021   Lateral Advancement Flap Technique   58 / 3.022   Cranial Advancement Flap Technique   59 / 3.023   Caudal Advancement Flap Technique   59 / 3.024   Rotation Flap Technique for Defects of Ala Nasi   59 / 3.025   Rotation Flap Technique for Defects of the Nasal Tip   61 / 3.026   Tunnel Flap Technique   61 / 3.027   Columella Nasi Reconstruction Technique   62 / 3.028   Island Flap Technique   62 / 3.029   Composite Grafts   62 / 3.030   Z-Flap Technique   63 / 3.031   Free Skin Grafting   63-/-3.032   Rhinophyma Therapy   63

3.033   Lips   64

3.034   Vermilionectomy for the Lower Lip (Langenbeck and von Bruns)   64 / 3.035   Triangular Excision   65 / 3.036   Advancement Flap Techniques for the Lower Lip (von Burow)   66 / 3.037   Lower Lip Repair (Estlander)   66 / 3.038   Transposition Flap Technique for Defects of the Lower Lip   67 / 3.039   VY-Flap Technique   67 / 3.040   Plastic Surgery to Widen the Mouth   68 / 3.041   Transposition Flap Technique for Upper Lip Repair   68 / 3.042   Advancement Flap Technique (von Burow) for Upper Lip Repair   68 / 3.043   Lower Lip Repair (Spiessl)   69 / 3.044   Surgical Therapy for Cheilitis Granulomatosa (Melkersson–Rosenthal Syndrome)   69 / 3.045   Correction of Thin Labium   70

3.046   Eyelids   70

3.047   Advancement Flap Technique (Inner Canthus)   70 / 3.048   Transposition Flap Technique (Inner Canthus)   71 / 3.049   Advancement–Rotation Flap Technique (Upper Eyelid)   71 / 3.050   Advancement Flap Technique (Lower Eyelid)   71 / 3.051   Rotation Flap Technique (Imre)   71 / 3.052   Transposition Flap Technique (Lower Eyelid)   72 / 3.053   Correction for Baggy Eyelids (Blepharoplasty)   72

3.054   Cheeks   75

3.055   Advancement Flap Technique   75 / 3.056   Transposition Flap Technique   75 / 3.057   Rotation Flap Technique   75

3.058   Auricle, Pre- and Postauriclar Region   75

3.059   Triangular Excision   75 / 3.060   Reduction Plasty of the Auricle (Trendelenburg)   76 / 3.061   Partial Amputation of the Auricle   76 / 3.062   Plastic Reconstruction of the Auricle for Partial Defects   79 / 3.063   Rotation Flap Technique   79 / 3.064   Transposition Flap Technique   79 / 3.065   Advancement Flap Technique   79 / 3.066   Tunnel Flap Technique   79 / 3.067   Chin, Throat, and Neck   79 / 3.068   Advancement Flap Technique   81 / 3.069   Rotation Flap Technique (Lateral Chin–Mandibular Area)   81 / 3.070   Rotation Flap Technique (Throat)   82 / 3.071   Double Rotation Flap Technique   82 / 3.072   Transposition Flap Technique   82

3.073   Trunk   83

3.074   Transposition Flap Technique   83 / 3.075   Rotation Flap Technique   83 /
3.076   Double Rotation Flap Technique   83 / 3.077   Free Skin Grafting Technique   83 /
3.078   Rehabilitation of Sagging Abdomen   84

3.079   Axilla   85

3.080   Transposition Flap Technique   85 / 3.081   Rotation Flap Technique   85 /
3.082   Surgical Therapy for Axillary Hyperhidrosis   85

3.083   Male Genital Region   85

3.084   Dorsal Incision   86 / 3.085   Circumcision   86 / 3.086   Phimosis Correction
(Rebreyoud [385])   87 / 3.087   Pedicled Flap Technique (Happle)   87 / 3.088   Amputation
of the Penis   88 / 3.089   Repair of a Defect in the Scrotal Area   88 / 3.090   Free Skin
Grafting Technique   88 / 3.091   Lymphangioplasty (Handley and Zieman [358, 570])   88 /
3.092   Testicular Biopsy   89 / 3.093   Surgery of Varicocele   89

3.094   Female Genital Region   90

3.095   Vulvectomy   90

3.096   Extremities   90

3.097   Multiple Z Flaps   90 / 3.098   Transposition Flap Technique   90 / 3.099   Free Skin
Grafting Technique   90 / 3.100   Surgical Therapy for Leg Ulcers   90

3.101   Hands and Feet   92

3.102   Free Skin Grafting Technique   92 / 3.103   Transposition Flap Technique   92 /
3.104   VY-Flap Technique   92 / 3.105   Multiple Z-Flap Technique   92 /
3.106   Dermabrasion   92 / 3.107   Nail Extraction   92 / 3.108   Nail Extraction Combined
with Triangular Excision   92 / 3.109   Triangular Excision (Emmet)   92 /

Bibliography   93

Index 111

Plates 119

Dermatosurgery

Introduction

The development of the specialty branches of medicine has not resulted from subclassification according to common aspects. Some branches are characterized according to certain organ systems, such as internal medicine, ophthalmology, otolaryngology, orthopedics, urology, or dermatology. A few are defined according to the methods applied (surgery, radiology); others are classified according to the patient's age (pediatrics, geriatrics), the exposition (internal medicine), or the pathogenic mechanisms; some limit themselves to certain illnesses. It is unavoidable and in many respects desirable that professional areas overlap. Two such overlapping specialties are surgery and dermatology. Although some surveys of the fringe area between surgery and dermatology [98, 99,396] have been made, a short introduction has been lacking.

In the interest of good patient care, specialties dealing with organ systems must comprise all possibilities of diagnosis, prevention, and therapy for the diseases of the organ concerned [430]. Operations on the skin are therefore as inseparable from dermatology as, for example, those on the inner ear are from otology. Some surgery is limited to the clinic, because of equipment and personnel requirements. However, the most frequently required operations can usually be carried out in the office. Unfortunately, these previously have not received adequate attention in dermatologic textbooks [476].

Minor operations, performed early, often avert major operations later. As a single organ, the skin is visible and accessible in its entirety, and consequently, it offers unique possibilities for the early detection and treatment of diseases. This is particularly true of tumors, which constitute the majority of surgical indications in dermatology. Even nonoperative tumor therapy requires minor surgery, e.g., a biopsy to confirm histologically the diagnosis. Treatment would rarely be justifiable in the absence of such confirmation [15,147,467].

Techniques suited for use in the office, such as punch biopsy, have been developed for this purpose [248,249, 364,488]. Rather than perform a biopsy, it is frequently more economical to remove immediately the focus radically [408].

1. Surgical Indications in Dermatology

1.001 Tumors, Preblastomatoses, Cysts, and Malformations

Benign and malignant neoplasms, as well as cancerous lesions and cysts, constitute the majority of skin conditions indicating surgery or biopsy. They will be grouped here according to tissue origin, and where possible we will list synonyms in common usage, the frequency of occurrence, the predilection sites, the margin of certainty to be expected from clinical diagnosis, and the differential diagnoses which must be frequently considered [147]. Afterwards, possible methods of treatment will be listed, and as necessary, improper procedures will also be mentioned.

1.002 Benign Epithelial Tumors

1.003 Basal Cell Papilloma. Verruca Seborrheica

Synonyms: seborrheic keratosis, verruca senilis.

This benign tumor, appearing predominantly on the trunk and head, is rare in children, but very common after age 40. Clinical diagnosis can be his-tologically confirmed in about 80% of cases.

Differential diagnosis: First, verruca vulgaris and less often, papillomatous nevus pigmentosus. Also Bowen's disease, actinic keratosis, squamous cell carcinoma, basal cell carcinoma and malignant melanoma. Contrary to popular opinion, of all basal cell papillomas presented for histologic examination, only 60% have already been diagnosed clinically [15,84]. More than 20% are thought to be papillomatous nevus pigmentosus, especially in younger patients.

Treatment of choice: removal with the curette.

Local anesthesia is often unnecessary [476], and if the curette is used skillfully, the specimen obtained can be used for histologic examination. This procedure is the least costly in terms of time and material, and the cosmetic result is optimal. If, however, a benign tumor is in an area unsuited for therapeutic curettage, such as the eyelids, scalpel excision under local anesthesia is recommended.

Although low-speed dermabrasion is possible (Sect. 2.30) [203], the magma produced cannot be histologically examined. Excision with the loop electrode requires even more time and material than with the curette.

Similarly, chemosurgery and X-ray therapy should be avoided because of unsatisfactory cosmetic results and the danger of after effects.

1.004. Verruca Vulgaris

Synonyms and variants: verruca plana, verruca filiformis, virus papilloma, plantar wart.

This occurs most frequently in areas exposed to virus, such as the hands, feet, and face. Virus warts are common to all age groups except newborn infants. About 60% of clinical diagnoses are confirmed histologically.

Differential diagnoses: verruca seborrhoica for older patients, as well as actinic keratosis and its carcinomas.

Treatment of choice: The location determines the treatment. For instance, after infiltration with a small amount of local anesthetic, filiform warts on the face can be lifted up with a forceps and removed with scalpel or scissors. The wound should be adapted well and closed with one or two fine interrupted sutures, which are left in for no more than one week and leave almost no scars. It is important that during the procedure no cells from the tumor-affected area are carried into the suture or the surrounding area.

However, on most areas of the body, virus warts are best treated with liquid nitrogen, applied with applicator sticks. After the wart and the surrounding area turn a whitish color, the wart either falls off within a few days or a blister-like elevation appears. If this does not occur, the procedure can be repeated. It is best not to apply too much liquid nitrogen initially since deep necrosis can result, leaving visible scars. This risk is even greater when using electro-desiccation, which requires that local anesthesia be administered carefully only on the area of the tumor. We recommend touching only the tip of the wart with the electric needle point so that necrosis affects only the viral parts of the tumor, since a disturbance of the surrounding area causes visible scarring.

In the case of plantar warts, it is best to remove the center of the wart by curettage after electrodesiccation of its periphery. Electrodesiccation alone would prolong the already lengthy healing process. If local anesthesia is used, the patient should be warned in advance that it is initially painful on the sole of the foot and may itch.

Other possible treatments for plantar warts are dabbing with nitric acid or applying a 60% salicylic acid plaster, cut exactly to the dimensions of the lesion and affixed with adhesive tape daily after bathing. It should remain in place for 24 h. If done properly, the necrotic tumor can be lifted out with the curette without local anesthesia, usually after 6–10 days. Commercially available wart tinctures are also sometimes effective. When the warts are below a nail, it is occasionally helpful to try Araviskij's nail removal method, i.e., applying a mixture of equal parts of potassium iodide and lanolin under plastic film for 8–14 days.

Even if there is no rapid spreading or no location warranting treatment, a spontaneous immunologically induced recurrence can be expected at any time [381]. This fact has probably helped to sustain the belief that warts can be psychotherapeutically influenced.

Warning: Do not use radiation therapy in view of the parity between its effectiveness and side effects [26,27].

1.005 Condyloma Acuminatum

Synonym: fig wart.

This virus-induced papilloma (similar to the verruca vulgaris) with little cornification appears on the epithelium of the genital and perianal region and occasionally in the oral cavity. It is common to all age groups except children. The clinical diagnosis is generally non-problematic. Unless there is excessive growth, squamous cell carcinoma may be excluded.

Treatment of choice: electrodesiccation under local or conduction anesthesia. Contact of only the tops of the condylomas limits their necrosis and keeps the surrounding skin intact, which promotes rapid healing. If the condyloma projections are extensive, we recommend Illig's procedure, i.e., electrodesiccation after which the cauterized tumors can be removed with a swab. Reepithelization results from applying an antibiotic ointment to these epidermal portions which are still intact. General anesthesia is necessary for larger affected areas and for the intraanal or intravaginal region. In order to treat even the slightest recurrence immediately, follow-ups should initially be conducted at weekly intervals; thus all neoplasms can be eradicated within a few weeks. A second possible treatment is the application of chemical agents (podophyllum).

1.006 Molluscum Contagiosum

Synonym: water wart.

Relatively common, especially among children, this is found primarily on the face, arms, hands, and feet.It is usually correctly diagnosed, except when occurring on the trunk or feet.

Differential diagnosis: sebaceous gland hyperplasia, basal cell carcinoma and plantar wart. The age group and location determine the diagnosis.

Treatment of choice: dab with antiseptic tincture, then slit with Moncorps' lancet and remove with a bent anatomic forceps. Anesthesia is generally unnecessary, but if the diagnosis is doubtful, excision under local anesthesia should be considered.

1.007 Verrucous Epidermal Nevus and Rare Epidermal Nevi

These benign epidermal tumors appear mostly on the head and trunk.

Treatment of choice: excision only, for they usually recur following curettage or dermabrasion.

1.008 Nevus Sebaceous (Jadassohn)

Rare, benign, appearing primarily on the head.

Differential diagnosis: nevus verrucosus, basal cell papilloma, possibly basal cell carcinoma.

Treatment of choice: excision only. The simultaneous occurrence of nevus sebaceus with basal cell carcinoma is rare.

1.009 Clear Cell Acanthoma (Degos)

Benign and rare, very seldom clinically diagnosed.

Treatment of choice: usually excision under another diagnosis. Other possible methods are curettage, dermabrasion, and K. Brehm's cantharidin blistering method [41].

1.010 Rare Benign Tumors of the Skin Glands

Synonyms and variants: Syringocystadenoma papilliferum, apocrine cystadenoma, eccrine spiradenoma, eccrine poroma, hydradenoma papilliferum, and benign mixed tumors.

Treatment of choice: only excision should be considered, although often treated under other diagnoses. In case of syringomas, it is usually neither necessary nor possible to remove all of them.

1.011 Sebaceous Gland Adenoma

Benign and rare, it usually appears on the head.

Treatment of choice: excision only.

1.012 Senile Sebaceous Gland Hyperplasia

This frequent, benign neoplasm is observed primarily on the head, especially the forehead, and is normally diagnosed clinically.

Differential diagnosis: basal amelanotic nevus.

Treatment of choice: excision or dermabrasion under local anesthesia.

1.013 Rhinophyma

Synonyms: hammer nose, potato nose.

Differential diagnosis: it is sometimes difficult to differentiate an accompanying basal carcinoma within the lesioned area.

Treatment of choice: decortication. This technique, described by von Hebra as early as 1881, consists of reconstructing the original shape of the nose according to old photographs of the patient [149,232].

1.014 Nevus Comedonicus

This benign and relatively rare neoplasm usually appears on the face in adults.

Differential diagnosis: possibly basal cell carcinoma or sebaceous gland hyperplasia.

Treatment of choice: excision only. Dermabrasion and curettage are not recommended, for after such therapy recurrences are frequent.

1.015 Trichofolliculoma

Synonym: hair follicle nevus.

This rare and benign tumor, which appears on the head, is seldom clinically diagnosed.

Differential diagnosis: nevus pigmentosus, cylindroma, epithelioma adenoides cysticum.

Treatment of choice: excision.

1.016 Malherbe's Epithelioma

Synonyms: calcifying epithelioma, pilomatrixoma.

This benign and faily common epithelioma was formerly often mistaken for an atheroma and excised without histologic examination. It is found especially in the shoulder girdle region, on the upper arm, and on the thigh, primarily in younger patients.

Differential diagnosis: follicle retention cysts or, in some cases, atheromas.

Treatment of choice: excision.

1.017 Cysts

Treatment of choice: excision in toto to prevent recurrence.

1.018 Follicle Retention Cysts

Synonyms and variants: atraumatic epidermal cysts, epidermoid cysts, atheroma.

Special type: steatocystomatosis multiplex (sebocystomatosis scroti).

Common except in children, these neoplasms occur especially on the head and trunk. The general term "follicle retention cysts" is preferred because tissue origin is often the same (although there is varying cell wall differentiation within the same cyst) and, with the exception of traumatic variants, the connection to a hair follicle can usually be observed if the correct incision is made. Clinical diagnosis is histologically verified in approximately 75% of all cases.

Differential diagnosis: nevi, histiocytomas, basal cell carcinomas, inflammatory granulomas, perifolliculitides. Malherbe's epithelioma is rare but is mistaken for a follicle retention cyst in approximately 75% of all cases.

Treatment of choice: total excision under local anethesia, and primary suturing. Electrodesiccation, recommended by Wilkinson for small cysts [507], is not suitable for every location and often leaves unsightly scars. Simple incision causes recurrences that are more difficult to treat.

1.019 Traumatic Epidermal Cysts

These are like follicle retention cysts (Sect. 1.018), except that they have no follicular connection to the skin surface.

Treatment of choice: Same as that for follicle retention cysts.

1.020 Milia

There are two varieties of milia: those appearing spontaneously in all age groups (these are relatively common, especially on the face) and those appearing after trauma, dermabrasion, split skin graft, and blistering (e.g., in the case of porphyria cutanea tarda or dermatitis herpetiformis soon after re-epithelization). After a short time, the latter variants usually gain access to the skin surface and disappear.

Treatment of choice: dab with antiseptic tincture, slit the surface with a lancet, and express.

1.021 Precanceroses

Only precancerous lesions in the stricter sense, such as actinic keratoses, are of special importance for dermatosurgery. Those lesions which are precancerous in the broader sense, such as farmer's skin and sailor's skin, cannot be treated surgically.

Treatment of choice: if possible, dermatosurgery. Warning: the oncogenic side effects of x-ray or chemotherapy in younger patients must be considered before deciding on either of these treatments.

1.022 Keratoma Solare

Synonyms: solar or actinic keratosis; keratoma "senile" or keratosis "senilis" are incorrect terms.

The predilection sites for precancerous lesions are in the stricter sense those surfaces exposed to sunlight (face, ears, back of hands, and front forearms). Keratoma solare, the most common precancerous lesion, occurs not only in older people with occupational exposure to sun ("farmer's skin"), but also in younger patients who have been exposed for many years to excessive amounts of natural or artificial sunlight [217].

Special types: keratosis solaris occurring in children suffering from xeroderma pigmentosum.

The clinical diagnosis is confirmed histologically in approximately 70% of all cases; in another 10%, carcinomas are discovered at the base of the original keratosis.

Differential diagnosis: basal cell carcinoma, verruca vulgaris, basal cell papilloma; and chondrodermatitis nodularis helicis chronica Winkler on the ear.

Treatment of choice: If cancer is suspected, excision is the only therapy. If cancer is not suspected treatment may be selected according to the location: excision, Schreus' zinc-chloride chemotherapy [435], Brehm's catharidin blistering method [39], or curettage. Other methods include X-ray therapy except for younger patients or those with xeroderma pigmentosum (the disadvantage of X-ray therapy is that the treatment and healing process is too long), local cytostatic therapy, carbon dioxide slush, and dermabrasion with rotary instruments [739,248,250,433, 434]. The use of vitamin A in treatment, mentioned in some of the literature on the subject, influences the symptom of hyperkeratosis more than it does the underlying precancerosis.

1.023 "Cornu Cutaneum." Compare Molluscum Contagiosum (Sect. 1.006)

Synonym: "cutaneous horn."

This is not a nosologic entity since different processes accompanying hyperkeratosis can be the cause. The most frequent is solar keratosis or a carcinoma on the base of an actinic keratoma, while verruca vulgaris or keratoacanthoma are somewhat less frequent.

Treatment of choice: excision [227].

1.024 Tar and Oil Keratoses

Synonym: pitch warts.

Premalignant and rare, they are found in the genital and forearm regions on turners and gem cutters who are exposed to oils containing chemical carcinogens and do not practice sufficient body hygiene.

Differential diagnosis: possibly arsenic keratoses if occurring in typical location.

Treatment of choice: excision under local anesthesia, especially if it is suspected that carcinogenesis has already begun. Other possible methods of treatment are the cantharidin blistering method, dermabrasion, or the loop electrode, the choice depending on the individual case.

Warning: In no case use X-ray treatment if the keratoses are located in the genital region.

1.025 Arsenic Keratosis

This is a type of precancerosis induced by arsenic which occurs on the stratum coreum of the palms and the soles of the feet. On other areas of the body it manifests itself more often as Bowen's disease. It is found especially among copper and nonferrous metal miners, but also among patients who either once worked with pesticides containing arsenic or took antipsoriatics containing it. A complete examination is necessary in order to rule out internal arsenic carcinomas.

Differential diagnosis: possibly callosities and palmoplantar keratoses.

Treatment of choice: excision. There is no alternative.

1.026 Bowen's Disease

This carcinoma in situ is relatively common, especially in older patients, and often appears after unobserved exposure to internal or external carcinogenic noxae, but can also develop from solar keratosis. The clinical diagnosis is histologically confirmed in only 40% of all cases. Almost another 10% consists of already manifest carcinomas.

Differential diagnosis: basal cell carcinomas and, in rare cases, basal cell papillomas.

Treatment of choice: If carcinogenesis is suspected, choose excision; if not, other possible methods are Brehm's cantharidin blistering method [39], Schreus' chemotherapy [435], X-ray therapy (see survey in Braun-Falco and Lukacs [38], dermabrasion [433], and local cytostatic treatment [179], depending on the disease's location. In each case, punch biopsy should be used before treatment to confirm histologically the diagnosis.

1.027 Erythroplasia of Queyrat

Premalignant and relatively rare, this counterpart to Bowen's disease is found on the mucous membrane of the cheeks and on the genitals.

Differential diagnosis: occasionally balanoposthitis, balanitis plasmocellularis (Zoon), etc.

Treatment of choice: excision; when occurring on genitals use material from the prepuce for plastic repair, according to Happle's method [187]. Further possibilities of therapy are cantharidin blistering method and X-ray.

1.028 Leukoplakia

Premalignant and relatively common, leukoplakia in the stricter sense is also a counterpart to Bowen's disease, occurring primarily in the oral cavity; it should be differentiated from leukoplakic conditions that are not precancerous.

Differential diagnosis: lichen planus, candidiasis, mucous plaques in connection with secondary syphilis, etc.

Special variant: leukoplakia of the lips, which can resemble actinic keratosis or a tar keratosis (see [217]. Its whitish color is caused by swollen stratum coreum and is common to all leukoplakic lesions.

Treatment of choice: excision, sometimes necessitating plastic surgery. However, if conditions are symptomatic and not precancerous, systemic treatment with vitamin A can be helpful. Neither treatment excludes the possibility of spontaneous recurrences.

1.029 Cheilitis Abrasiva Precancerosa (Manganotti)

This is a special type of actinic leukoplakia (Sect. 1.028).

Treatment of choice: same as that for leukoplakia, e.g., excision using vermilionectomy [323].

1.030 Radiodermatitis, Roentgenism

This is a precancerosis in the broader sense which is becoming less common, due to the increased use of plastic surgery in therapy.

Treatment of choice: excision only [355]. When necessary, plastic replacement of X-ray-damaged tissue ensures a complete cure.

1.031 Lichen Sclerosus et Atrophicans

Synonyms and variants: When occurring on the trunk, "white spot disease"; on the genitals, kraurosis vulvae in the female or balanoposthitis sclerotica obliterans Stühmer in the male. This is said to be a precancerosis in the broader sense.

Treatment of choice: excision; in males, circumcision. Further possibilities of therapy are dermabrasion (see [138,139]) and intralesional and topical corticosteroid application.

1.032 Intraepidermal Epithelioma (Borst-Jadassohn)

Often an early stage in the development of Bowen's disease, this is rarely diagnosed clinically and is therefore excised under other diagnoses.

1.033 Carcinomas

These malignant, metastasizing epithelial tumors occupy a special position in general oncology, for they are visible and accessible, two features frequently leading to an early diagnosis with prompt treatment and therefore excellent prospects of a complete cure.

1.034 Squamous Cell Carcinoma

Synonym: prickle cell carcinoma. This is "skin cancer" in the stricter sense.

Especially frequent in elderly patients, this is the most common malignant metastasizing tumor occurring on skin areas exposed to the sun's ultraviolet rays. About two-thirds of clinical diagnoses are confirmed histologically.

Differential diagnosis: basal cell carcinomas, solar keratosis without carcinomatous growth, and keratoacanthoma are frequent; less common are basal cell papillomas, postinflammatory alterations, scars, Morbus Bowen, and reactive epidermal hyperplasia.

The varying grades I–IV and special varieties like the Bowen carcinoma, epithelioma mixtum, and others, are defined according to histologic differentiation and cornification.

Treatment of choice: excision as soon as possible. If a simple excision is no longer possible, plastic surgery must be performed. If metastases to the regional lymph nodes are suspected, en bloc excision is necessary. Further possibilities of therapy are radiation after the diagnosis is confirmed histologically by biopsy. However, "posttreatment" radiation following total excision must not be used since it only injures the remaining tissue and has detrimental after effects. Besides radiation Moh's chemotherapy [303] should be considered [47] if the tumors are difficult to reach. Cytostatic chemotherapy should be regarded only as a palliation.

1.035 Carcinomas of the Skin Appendages

These uncommon tumors are rarely diagnosed clinically.

Treatment of choice: the same as for squamous cell carcinoma (Sect. 1.34) of the superficial epithelium.

1.036 Paget Carcinoma

Synonym: Paget's disease of the nipple. Although occasionally listed in abstracts as a precancerosis, the Paget carcinoma is an intraepithelial carcinoma of the lactiferous ducts in the nipple areola.

Special form: a rare extramammary Paget's disease in areas with apocrine glands.

Differential diagnosis: eczema of the nipple areola.

Treatment of choice: punch biopsy immediately following the first consultation to ensure correct diagnosis. Radical surgical removal should be performed as soon as possible after the diagnosis is histologically confirmed.

1.037 Skin Metastases of Internal Carcinomas

These are usually diagnosed clinically after the primary tumor has already been discovered.

Treatment of choice: excision, X-ray, or, where appropriate, chemotherapy as a palliative measure.

1.038 Pseudocancerous Lesions

These are a heterogeneous group of tumors and reactive hyperplastic neoplasms with a favorable prognosis.

1.039 Keratoacanthoma

Synonyms: molluscum pseudocarcinomatosum, molluscum sebaceum, and acanthokeratoma.

Special varieties: aggregated keratoacanthomas and multiple keratoacanthomas. This pseudocarcinomatous tumor of the hair follicle is characterized by infiltrative growth, lack of metastasis, and spontaneous involution. It is roughly one third as common as squamous cell carcinoma and initially is diagnosed histologically in one out of ten cases. It appears most frequently in older patients on skin areas exposed to sunlight. The clinical diagnosis is confirmed histologically in about 75% of all cases.

Differential diagnosis: squamous cell carcinomas, basal cell carcinomas, and common warts [180].

Treatment of choice: excision. One cannot rely on spontaneous involution since neither its onset nor the present extent of the destruction can be predicted. Furthermore, scars left from spontaneous involution, like those from radiation therapy, are aesthetically unsatisfying. Only by a transverse incision through the entire tumor can the diagnosis be histologically verified. A less than total excision results in rapid recurrence [164].

1.040 Papillomatosis Cutis Carcinoides Gottron

This pseudomalignancy always arises on a predamaged skin area, such as a chronic leg ulcer.

Treatment of choice: excision. The papillomatosis can be radically removed and the surgical defect covered by split-thickness or even full-thickness skin graft. If there is recurrence, additional cytostatic drugs must be applied locally and or systematically [356].

1.041 Pseudocarcinomous Hyperplasia

This develops in chronic ulcers, radiodermatitis, and inflammatory or tumorous lesions.

Treatment of choice: excision, if malignancy is suspected or in order to rule it out.

1.042 Oral Florid Papillomatosis

Synonym: carcinoid mucosal papillomatosis. *Treatment of choice:* excision of the involved area, frequently because of a suspected carcinoma. Kryosurgery is possible too. Systemic cytostatic therapy may be necessary in the case of inoperable recurrences.

1.043 Basal Cell Carcinoma and Related Tumors

These are primarily semimalignant, epithelial tumors, ranging from barely destructive to highly destructive local neoplasms that rarely metastasize and never originate from precanceroses in the stricter sense (cf. survey in [170], [218]). Their variants occur as differentiations within a tumor or as different tumors on the same patient as in the case of genetically determined basaliomatoses. Therefore we group them together. Morphologically identical tumors occur in multiple forms as symptoms of certain syndromes that frequently afflict younger patients.

1.044 Basal Cell Carcinoma

Synonym: basal cell epithelioma.

Because it does not as a rule metastasize, the ordinary induced basal cell carcinoma is a so-called semimalignant tumor. It occurs in older patients primarily on skin that has been damaged by sunlight. It is second in frequency of all skin tumors. About one fifth of all routine initial tests in dermatohistopathologic laboratories involve cases that were diagnosed clinically as basal cell carcinoma and which are verified in roughly 75% of all cases.

Differential diagnosis: squamous cell carcinoma, solar actinic keratosis with nodular actinic elastosis, basal cell papillomas, keratoacanthomas (briefer anamnesis), nevus pigmentosus, and Bowen's disease (especially the superficially spreading forms). The presence of nodular, solid, or cystic types of neoplasm facilitates the delimitation of the tumor; this is important for therapy, because tumor growth is not believed to extend beyond the nodules, which are visibly suffused by telangiectasia. Similarly, the thread-like papular margin around the edge demarcates the actual limit of the largely superficial tumor growth in the basal cell carcinoma of the trunk. On the other hand, it is often difficult to determine the edge of the tumor in cases like "ulcus rodens" and "epithelioma planum et cicatricans," those tumors that spread like scleroderma and the extreme form of the "ulcus terebrans." Moreover, one should expect tumor components which undermine the area but are not visible, especially in the scalp area. In planning the excision, an intraoperative frozen section of the incision's edges should be considered.

Treatment of choice: excision and if extent and location require it, either plastic repairs of the defect, or Moh's chemosurgery [302,303] [47]. While Schreus' zincchloride chemotherapy is often effective for small foci [435], in older patients and on appropriate locations, X-ray therapy may be preferable [38]. Treatment that employs electrocauterization or, in some cases, electrodesiccation and curettage [103] usually leads to unsatisfying cosmetic results and therefore should be considered only in those cases where this aspect can be totally ignored.

Naturally, before administering the proposed therapies, as well as topical cytostatic treatment of basal cell carcinomas [179] (the extent of which are difficult to determine), the diagnosis must be verified histologically. X-ray therapy must be absolutely rejected for younger patients. Aftereffects of radiation include X-ray-induced basal cell carcinomas. However, when in doubt, radical surgery is always preferable. Defects which cannot be repaired are often sufficiently corrected by prostheses [80].

1.045 Premalignant Fibroepithelial Tumor (Pinkus)

This tumor seldom occurs and is easily mistaken for a fibroma or nevus in clinical diagnoses.

Treatment of choice: excision (often under another clinical diagnosis). Practically no other treatment is possible, above all no X-ray therapy since this tumor is reported to occur on skin damaged by radiation.

1.046 Spiegler's Tumor

Synonym: dermal cylindroma.

This relatively uncommon suborganoid hamartoma occurs primarily on the scalp and its incidence increases with age.

Differential diagnosis: follicle retention cysts or, in some cases, atheromas, and nevus pigmentosus.

Treatment of choice: excision. Alternative treatments are unsatisfactory.

1.047 Epithelioma Adenoids Cysticum (Brooke)

Synonym: trichoepithelioma.

Relatively less common than Spiegler's tumor, this occurs in different forms at the root of the nose, on the nasolabial creases, and the cheeks.

Treatment of choice: excision and possible plastic replacement of affected skin areas where there are multiple lesions. Other treatments do not prove satisfactory.

1.048 Nevoid Basal Cell Carcinomas

Synonym: phacomatosis Brooke-Spiegler.

This is a combination to varying degrees of Spiegler's tumor (Sects. 1.046 and 1.047) and basal cell carcinomas of other forms (Sect. 1.044), which occurs among patients as an autosomal dominant disease.

Treatment of choice: depends on the kind of tumor present. However, before using X-ray therapy, the age of the patient and the possibility that X-rays may induce additional basal cell carcinomas by ionizing rays must be considered.

1.049 Basal Cell Nevus Syndrome (Fifth Phacomatosis)

Synonyms: nevoid basal cell carcinomas, 5th phacomatosis, and basal cell nevus syndrome.

This is also a rare hereditary disease of autosomal dominance usually beginning during childhood and occurring with basal cell carcinomas of all kinds, some of which are slow-spreading initially (basal cell nevus) and some of which have numerous nevi pigmentosi. It is often accompanied by jaw cysts, split ribs, and varied skeletal malformations primarily of the spine and the central nervous system, such as agenesis of the callous corpus, calcifications of the falx of the cerebrum, etc., and pitted-looking keratoses on the palms and soles of the feet.

Treatment of choice: same as for phacomatosis (Brooke-Spiegler) mentioned above.

1.050 Benign Tumors of the Pigment-Producing Cells

Since the definition of a "tumor," as with cysts, is to some extent problematic, it is our intention to present a pragmatic survey rather than a perfect classifying system.

1.051 Lentigo

Synonym: freckle.

Especially common on the face, it is rarely excised for cosmetic reasons or because a premalignant or malignant growth is suspected.

Differential diagnosis: nevus pigmentosus (which can possibly result from a lentigo), in some cases, lentigo maligna (Dubreuilh) or superficial spreading melanoma.

Treatment of choice: excision or planing with rotary instruments, allowing for the fact that pigment is also found in the upper corium.

1.052 Lentigo Senilis

This benign tumor is often found on the back of the hands and face of older patients who have had long exposure to sun; yet it is seldom treated.

Differential diagnosis: lentigo maligna (Dubreuilh), lentigo maligna melanoma; also flat basal cell papillomas, and, in some case, pigmented solar keratoses.

Treatment of choice: excision under local anesthesia or dermabrasion with rotary instruments, considering that pigment has trickled down into the upper corium as well, as is the case for tar and oil keratoses (Sect. 1.024), but also ensuring that the skin relief is not severely flattened.

1.053 Nevus Pigmentosus

Synonyms and variations: "mole," "pigmented-mole," in some cases, "nevus papillomatosus," and "pilosus."

Special form: Sutton's halo nevus or hairy nevus (Sect. 1.056).

This is the most common skin tumor, occurring on the trunk and the head, especially between ages 20 and 40. The clinical diagnosis is histologically verified in over 80% of all cases.

Differential diagnosis: basal cell papilloma, for papillomatous types; lentigo, histiocytoma, and basal cell carcinoma for corial forms. The continued junctional activity of the mole and its tendency to grow can be expected among younger patients and those having darker pigmentation. Among older patients and those of light pigmentation, further reduction of the pigment content is more likely; however, the mole will not regress. The belief, still frequently encountered in surgical literature, that common nevus pigmentosis should not be treated because of the purported danger of cancer has absolutely no basis in fact [157,225].

Treatment of choice: excision, during which not only the nevus itself (papillomatous types usually project less deeply than nonpapillomatous types) is completely excised, but also all hair follicles within the nevus. Therefore the incision must be made vertically into the deepest layer of tissue but never in cuneiform shape. The tissue is separated in the subcutis below the hair follicles, which are usually more darkly pigmented and thicker than the hair of the surrounding area. There is always the danger that hairs from a separated follicle will grow out again, boring through the fresh scar and causing a foreign body reaction, which has unsatisfactory cosmetic results. In the case of Sutton's nevus, instead of excising the entire halo, an alternative is simply to wait since the halo's formation signals an immunity response to the tumor which can result in its spontaneous regression. Curettage is not possible in papillomatous cases either, due to the high content of connective tissue.

Likewise, x-ray therapy should be regarded as unacceptable in view of its aftereffects.

1.054 Juvenile Melanoma (Spitz)

Synonyms: spindle cell nevus, Spitz tumor.

This is a benign, relatively uncommon tumor occurring primarily on the face of young patients.

Differential diagnosis: forms of nevi and angiomas.

Treatment of choice: excision.

1.055 Nevus Coeruleus

Synonym: blue nevus.

Special types include the multicellular varieties such as neuroid nevus bleu Masson or, in some cases, cellular blue nevus Allen. The clinical diagnosis of this uncommon tumor has a high rate of accuracy.

Differential diagnosis: histiocytoma and basal cell carcinoma.

Treatment of choice: excision.

1.056 Nevus Pilosus

Synonym: hairy mole.

When this uncommon neoplasm is microscopically examined, the findings are similar to those for nevus pigmen-

tosus (Sect. 1.053) with the differences that 1) the hairy mole is present from birth, whereas normal nevi first appear during childhood and adolescence, and 2) it frequently spreads over a large area.

Treatment of choice: excision, often requiring plastic repair of the defect, depending on the location or repetition of the treatments.

1.057 Melanophacomatosis (Virchow-Rokitansky-Touraine)

Synonym: neurocutaneous melanoblastosis.

This is a malformation syndrome characterized by extensive hairy nevi and growing nevi pigmentosi and pilosi present from birth. In this type of phacomatosis, malignant melanomas occur relatively frequently in the skin or central nervous system even among young patients. These in turn must be classified as a special type of malignant melanoma apart from those distinguished by Clark et al. [54] and listed in Section 1.058.

Treatment of choice (and prophylaxis): extended and usually repeated excision, although plastic repair is in some cases very difficult.

1.058 Premalignant and Malignant Neogenesis of the Pigment-Producing Cells (Steigleder and Clark et al. [54,466])

1.059 Lentigo Maligna, Premalignant Melanosis Dubreuilh

Synonym: lentigo maligna Hutchinson.

This is a premalignant, relatively uncommon neoplasm occurring in older patients on areas of skin exposed to sunlight (e.g., the face). Sunlight acts as the "promotor," not the initiator, of malignancy in this disease [503].

Differential diagnosis: superficial spreading melanoma, lentigo senilis, and, for instance, in individual cases where there is light pigmentation, Bowen's disease as well [detailed surveys in 229,425,469].

Treatment of choice: excision and X-ray therapy. Other possible treatments are dermabrasion, cauterizaton, and local chemotherapy [e.g., 433,434]. However, before proceeding with any treatment other than excision, the diagnosis should be confirmed histologically to rule out superficial spreading melanoma, which is often difficult to differentiate clinically.

Warning: A delay in treatment can mean the development of a harmful melanoma.

1.060 Lentigo Maligna Melanoma, Dubreuilh Melanoma

This is a nodular tumor which develops within a "lentigo maligna" at any time after the onset of this disease.

Differential diagnosis: the more common superficial spreading melanoma with secondary nodular formation.

Treatment of choice: the same as that for the other types of melanomas.

1.061 Superficial Spreading Melanoma

This melanoma spreads first intraepidermally over an area, especially on the trunk in men or extremities in women. Present opinion is that the prognosis is not essentially better than for nodular melanoma once vertical growth has begun [survey:190,277,228]. It depends on the level of invasion [54] and tumor thickness [40,489,490]. Invasion exceeding level 3 and a thickness more than 1.5 mm deteriorate the prognosis.

Differential diagnosis: depending on location, lentigo maligna, lentigo maligna melanoma, lentigo senilis, and flat basal cell papillomas. The majority of neoplasms formerly diagnosed as Dubreuilh melanoma in areas not exposed to sunlight would today probably be classified as superficial spreading melanomas [227,228,229,297,342,347]. The slightest irregularities in the skin relief may signal that vertical growth has already begun [211].

Treatment of choice: excision far into the healthy tissue (5 cm, 2 in.), a procedure similar in principle to that for nodular melanoma.

1.062 Nodular Malignant Melanoma

This prognostically unfavorable malignant tumor is not too rare. "Melanoma" is the clinical diagnosis in about 1% of all routine entries presented for dermatohistologic examination.

Differential diagnosis: Considerably more difficult than for other types of melanomas, diagnosis is verified in about half of all cases. Conversely, less than 60% of all nodular melanomas which were discovered histologically were already recognized clinically, in contrast to 75% for other types of melanomas [147]. It is relatively common for nevus pigmentosus to be misdiagnosed as nodular melanomas, less often as basal cell papillomas, hemangiomas, blue nevi, juvenile melanomas, basal cell carcinomas, scars, cysts, or histiocytomas.

Melanomas generally can, on the other hand, hide behind a variety of clinical diagnoses [228,231]: hemangiomas, nevus pigmentosus, basal cell papillomas, lentigo maligna, Bowen's disease, squamous cell carcinomas, and histiocytomas.

Treatment of choice: when detected early or in initial stage, excision into the healthy tissue up to the fascia with a 2-in. safety margin [333]. According to statistics, more radical measures do not necessarily improve the chances for cure or survival [788]. However, some researchers' findings [59,377] suggest a prophylactic advantage in simultaneously extirpating the regional lymph nodes when tumor location suggests it, for they are just as frequently affected when the clinical findings do not indicate metastases as when they do [494]. (Therefore a purely clinical division of the disease's stages is open to question.) Only in cases of close proximity of the two does the en bloc extirpation of the tumor and lymph nodes seem to be more advantageous than removal in separate operations [458]. The problem in judging the success of all procedures up to now has been the lack of extensive postoperative observation periods on greater numbers of patients, a prerequisite for any statistical evaluation [190,229]. This also applies for the present to the combination of local excision and endolymphatic therapy [89,90, 230,495].

Lately, one of the more radical treatments that seems to offer the patient am improved chance [279] is excision combined with either therapeutic resection of the lymph node block or closed-circuit hyperthermic perfusion of the affected extremities with large doses of special cytotoxic agents such as phenylalanine mustard (cf. survey in [432]).

Since this procedure can be performed only in a few centers, it is evident that cooperation with a hospital is required for the necessary continual and frequent check-ups.

During stage II, depending on the requirements imposed by location, additional radical procedures are instituted which, in some cases, take the form of closed-circuit perfusion. Extensive amputations should be considered only if technically necessary (for instance, necrosis following perfusion), for they worsen the patient's overall condition and lessen his chances [333].

During stage III, local excision of the operable metastases is still usually preferred, on the assumption that the immunologic defense mechanism is improved by reducing the tumor's total mass. However, especially in this connection, cryosurgical destruction of the nodes and their retention in situ must likewise be considered. And because the immunologic defense system is important for the course of the therapy, systemic cytotoxic treatment must currently be avoided if at all possible, while any other treatment which would activate the cellular immunologic defense should be used as supportive therapy during all stages [277,280, 469,494].

1.063 Benign Tumors and Pseudotumors of the Connective Tissues

1.064 Histiocytoma, Dermatofibroma

Synonyms and variants: nodulus cutaneus Arning-Lewandrowsky, dermatofibroma lenticulare Schreus, nodular subepidermal fibrosis Michelson, sclerosing anginoma Gros-Wolbach, and others.

Some of the various forms have been described as independent diseases, but today they are felt to represent different variants or stages of development of the same, probably recurring, benign neoplasm (survey in [84]). The histiocytoma is the most common connective-tissue skin tumor of the extremities in patients aged 20-50 and occurs as the eighth most frequent initial diagnosis during routine dermatohistopathologic examination.

Although the clinical diagnosis is almost always verified, a certain proportion of histiocytomas are not diagnosed clinically in the primary stage and are mistaken for nevus pigmentosus, basal cell carcinomas, follicular retention cysts, foreign body granulomas, blue nevi, and others.

Treatment of choice: excision. No other treatment is possible, although occasionally, flattening and reduction of the hemosiderin pigmentation may occur by itself.

1.065 Nevoxanthoendothelioma

Synonyms: juvenile xanthogranuloma, juvenile xanthoma, and nevoxanthoma.

This rare, benign histiocytic tumor can occur anywhere on the body within the first few months after birth. Initial rapid growth is followed by arrest and usually spontaneous involution after approximately 1 year.

Differential diagnosis: In spite of the tumor's characteristic syndrome, it is occasionally difficult to differentiate from a sarcoma.

Treatment of choice: generally waiting for its spontaneous involution, unless the diagnosis is doubtful, in which case an excision should be made.

Warning: partial excision without correct closure of the wound should be avoided in all cases due to the danger of disfiguring scarring.

1.066 Xanthelasmas

These are lesions which usually occur on the upper eyelid and at the eye's inner corner, frequently among middle-aged women.

Differential diagnosis: difficult only in its differentiation from a basal cell carcinoma in atypical cases.

Treatment of choice: excision, if therapy is desired.

Warning: Scarring is very likely to result.

1.067 Xantomas

Xantomas appear most commonly due to dysfunctions of the lipometabolism, especially on the extensor surface of the small and large joints.

Differential diagnosis: simple.

Treatment of choice: Single foci that cause functional or cosmetic impairment can be excised, but the basic internal disease must be treated additionally.

1.068 Keloid

This common reactive tumor of the connective tissue caused by certain noxae (such as burns or in some cases, scalding, vaccination, or the intrusion of foreign bodies) occurs especially during childhood and foremost in certain skin regions such as the ear lobes, mouth, chin, chest, and shoulder area in persons who are predisposed to it. A familiar tendency is observed especially among some non-Caucasion population groups [403].

Differential diagnosis: frequently

shows so-called "spontaneous" keloids to result from foreign body granulomas (sand, safety glass, glove powder, suture material), but cannot strictly delimit keloids from hypertrophic scars [404].

Treatment of choice: the procedure depends on the size and age of the tumor as well as the individual's complaints [38]. Excision alone is problematic because of the danger of recurrence. If the focus is small and not older than six months, radiation or injections of glucocorticoid [138] can be considered, but larger or older keloids must be excised. As soon as there are signs of renewed keloid or hypertrophic scarring, injections of glucocorticoid crystal suspension and possibly radiation treatments should be given.

1.069 Hypertrophic Scars

The differences between hypertrophic scars and the keloid, as stated above, are not strictly defined [403, 404].

Treatment of choice: the same conservative measures applicable to the keloid [137], as well as topical application of corticoid.

1.070 Pseudosarcomatous Fasciitis

Synonyms: fasciitis nodularis and proliferative subcutaneous fasciitis.

These rare pseudotumorous lesions occur among the middle-aged and the elderly.

Differential diagnosis: due to the rapid spread of the nodes, they are difficult to differentiate clinically from dermatofibrosarcoma protuberans or a sarcoma.

Treatment of choice: complete excision of the focus.

1.071 Desmoid Tumor

Synonym: desmona.

Rare and benign, this tumor frequently reoccurs in the subumbilical paramedian region among women who have borne several children.

Treatment of choice: excision.

1.072 Nontumorous Fibroplasia (see Sect. 1.117)

1.073 Adenoma Sebaceum in Conjunction with Phacomatosis (Bourneville-Pringle)

These characteristic tiny fibromatous nodules are found in the centrofacial area.

Treatment of choice: occasionally the object of cosmetic correction for reasons of social acceptance, they can be smoothed down by skin planing, although new nodules will recur with time.

1.074 Semimalignant and Malignant Tumors of the Connective Tissue

1.075 Dermatofibrosarcoma Protuberans

Rare and semimalignant, this tumor of the skin's connective tissue occurs predominantly on the trunk.

Differential diagnosis: at onset, sometimes incorrectly diagnosed as a histiocytoma or a basal cell carcinoma.

Treatment of choice: excision far into the healthy tissue.

1.076 Fibrosarcoma

This malignant tumor occurs among all age groups.

Differential diagnosis: first differentiate from a histiocytoma or dermatofibrosarcoma protuberans and sometimes from a basal cell carcinoma or malignant melanoma.

Treatment of choice: radical excision.

1.077 Other Sarcomatous Forms

Treatment of choice: excision, if sarcomas of the skin are both highly fibrous and sharply differentiated. The less this is so, the more expedient are radiation and polycytostatic therapy.

1.078 Tumors of the Fatty Tissue

Only the relatively common, benign tumors are of practical interest to the dermatologist.

1.079 Lipoma

Special form: angiolipoma.
These tumors occur relatively seldom on the trunk and the extremities of middle-aged patients.

Differential diagnosis: sometimes difficult to differentiate from cysts (Sect. 1.018 and 1.019).

Treatment of choice: excision.

1.080 Lipomatosis Dolorosa

Lipomatous nodes occur in multiple forms, some of which are sensitive to pressure.

Treatment of choice: excision of the most disturbing nodes.

1.081 Benign Lymphoplasias of the Skin

1.082 Lymphocytoma Cutis

Synonym: lymphadenosis cutis benigna Baefverstedt.

This relatively rare, benign tumor occurs especially on the face or ear lobe in all age groups.

Differential diagnosis: depending on the location and patient's age, histiocytoma, mastocytoma faciale, or sarcoidosis.

Treatment of choice: if spontaneous involution fails to occur, penicillin; if that is ineffective, X-ray therapy. Excision should be resorted to only under three conditions: inadequate response to conservative therapy, diagnostic uncertainty, or the fact that excision will conclude therapy in the shortest time.

1.083 Malignant Lymphomas and Hemoblastoses

To verify histologically the diagnosis of mycosis fungoides (Alibert-Bazin), or of cutaneous foci of malignant lymphogranulomatosis (Paltauf-Sternberg-Hodgkin), or of malignant "reticuloses," of the "reticulosarcomatosis" (Gottron), or the "reticulum cell sarcomatoses" and hemoblastoses, or to control the course of the disease during treatment, individual foci are excised.

Treatment of choice: application of cytostatics and X-ray therapy [38], in cooperation with the hematologist.

1.084 Benign Tumors of the Vascular and Smooth Muscle Systems

1.085 Eruptive Angioma

Synonyms: granuloma teleangiectaticum, granuloma pediculatum, and erroneously [328] "granuloma pyogenicum."

Common in all age groups and in any location, its diagnosis is confirmed histologically in roughly 75% of all cases.

Differential diagnosis: sometimes difficult to differentiate from squamous cell carcinoma, basal cell carcinoma, basal cell papilloma, histiocytoma, keratoacanthoma, nevus pigmentosus, or malignant melanoma [147].

Treatment of choice: total excision, otherwise danger of recurrence. Nonsurgical treatment is not advisable without histologic verification of the diagnoses listed.

1.086 Angioma Senile

Synonym: senile angiectasia.

Commonly occurring on the trunk of elderly people this neoplasm begins as a proliferating benign hemangioma, which ceases spontaneously after a period of growth and leaves behind as a final stage a tumor structure consisting solely of distended capillaries without capillary branches [426].

Differential diagnosis: unproblematic.

Treatment of choice: usually unnecessary. If the neoplasm is bleeding and in a location where minor injuries are likely to occur or if it detracts cosmetically, then either excision or treatment with diathermy is recommended.

1.087 Nevus Araneus

Synonym: spider nevus.

Common on the face and extremities of younger patients, it should not be mistaken for Eppinger's "liver stars."

Treatment of choice: sclerosation of the central vessel with diathermy. Anesthesia is generally unnecessary.

1.088 Angiokeratoma. (Preferable [231]: thrombosed angioma.)

Variants: angiokeratoma neviforme,

angiokeratoma in Fabry's disease, and angioma verrucosum. The neoplasm is fairly common and appears in all body areas.

Differential diagnosis: may sometimes be difficult to rule out a malignant melanoma when single tumors occur in elderly persons [231].

Treatment of choice: excision or electrodesiccation.

Warning: If a malignant melanoma is suspected, perform a frozen section for immediate histologic examination.

1.089 Angiokeratoma Akroasphyticum Mibelli

This rare hereditary lesion occurs in multiple forms, especially on the dorsal surface of the fingers and toes in children before puberty.

Treatment of choice: diathermy.

1.090 Angiokeratoma Inpunctiforme Scroti s. Vulvae Fordyce

This is a relatively common lesion, especially among the elderly.

Differential diagnosis: the possibility of the rare and prognostically more serious Fabry's disease should be considered.

Treatment of choice: usually unnecessary, but possible with diathermy.

1.091 Fabry's Disease

Angiokeratotic skin lesions represent only one of the many symptoms of this hereditary skin disease.

Treatment of choice: operative measures usually limited to biopsies.

1.092 Capillary Hemangioma

Synonyms: "strawberry angioma" and hemangioma simplex.

Variants: eruptive angioma (Sect. 1.085) and angioma "senile" (Sect. 1.086).

The most common forms are plano-tuberous and tuberonodular angiomas in infancy, which are seldom clearly differentiated from cavernous hemangiomas (Sect. 1.093). The angiomas of infancy undergo spontaneous involution in the majority of cases during the first years.

Treatment of choice: as long as a focus is very small, it can easily be excised without any aftereffects. However, if spontaneous involution fails to take place or if the initial growth causes alarm, beta-ray therapy should be considered because beta rays often seem to stimulate further spontaneous involution. Also, they provide an alternative to the risks of deeper-reaching soft radiation on infants and toddlers [cf. 222].

1.093 Cavernous Hemangioma

This rare tumor, occasionally observed in all age groups and on all skin areas, does not undergo substantial spontaneous involution (arterial or venous cavernomas [209,427]).

Differential diagnosis: distinguishable from capillary hemangioma by its deeper location and the wall structure of connective muscle tissue in its vascular components.

Treatment of choice: excision. In contrast to the planotuberous capillary hemangiomas, this type is neither very sensitive to radiation nor is it influenced by beta rays, due primarily to its deepseated location.

1.094 Glomus Tumor

Synonyms: angiomyoneuroma and glomangioma.

This tumor has solid and more cavernous forms, the latter causing little difficulty. They are relatively uncommon and occur primarily before puberty, especially on the extremities.

Differential diagnosis: sometimes difficult to differentiate from leiomyoma and blue nevus.

Treatment of choice: excision.

1.095 Multiple Familial Glomus Tumors

This dermatosis, as an autosomal dominant disease is not combined with any other lesions. Cavernous forms, which are not painful to the touch, predominate.

Treatment of choice: none or excision.

1.096 Leiomyoma, Angioleiomyoma

These rare, benign tumors, appearing especially in multiple forms, extend mainly from the musculi arrectores pilorum or the vascular walls.

Differential diagnosis: when sensitive to pressure, they are difficult to differentiate from glomus tumors.

Treatment of choice: only excision.

1.097 Granular Cell Myoblastoma

The tissue origin of this very rare tumor, usually occurring among middle-aged patients, is still a controversial matter. Possibly, it is a reactive growth. In most cases the diagnosis is done histologically.

Treatment of choice: only excision.

1.098 Lymphangiomas

These very rare tumors are divided into circumscript, superficial, and deep cavernous forms.

Treatment of choice: the factors in each individual case must be carefully weighed. If the tumor lies very deep, surgery is difficult; although it is only slightly sensitive to radiation, betatron therapy should be attempted. Otherwise, excision in suitable cases is recommended.

1.099 Vascular Nevi

1.100 Nevus Teleangiectaticus Lateralis

Synonyms: nevus flammeus and nevus vinosus.

This is a relatively rare congenital malformation with increased and dilated capillaries circumscribed within the corium. In monographs on pathology, this lesion is commonly confused [216,232a]. When it occurs, as it frequently does, in a segmental arrangement on the face one must weigh the possibility of its being a symptom of a nevus flammeus and Sturge-Weber syndrome.

Treatment of choice: correction by plastic surgery is sometimes possible.

Warning: Radiation therapy and carbon dioxide slush, previously recommended in some cases, should never be used since they may considerably worsen the condition.

1.101 Nevus Flammeus Medialis Unna

Synonym: "Unna's pale teleangiectatic nevus."

This is similar to nevus telegiangiectaticus (Sect. 1.100) but is located in the middle of the forehead or neck and usually pales gradually on its own accord.

Treatment of choice: no therapy.

1.102 Semimalignant and Malignant Vascular Tumors

1.103 Hemangiopericytoma

This extremely rare and seldom clinically diagnosed tumor is observed on the trunk and head in all age groups.

Treatment of choice: since it is only slightly sensitive to radiation, excision far into the healthy tissue is the only possible therapy.

1.104 Hemangioendothelioma

This very rare tumor exhibits different variants. It occurs more frequently in older patients than in children.

Treatment of choice: radical excision where possible or radiation therapy where not; radiation therapy is more likely to be effective for hemangioendothelioma, according to Braun-Falco [28], than for hemangiopericytoma.

1.105 Kaposi's Sarcoma

This tumor of the extremities, especially the lower ones, often arises multicentrically.

Differential diagnosis: sometimes foreign body granulomas have a similar appearance to this neoplasm in its primary stages.

Treatment of choice: excision as well as radiation therapy are effective, but only on neoplasms that have not spread much. Later, perfusion therapy may be possible, as in the treatment of malignant melanoma.

1.106 Hemangiosarcoma

This is a rare, malignant tumor.

Treatment of choice: only an early and radical surgical removal.

1.107 Tumors of the Nerves and Nerve Sheaths

These are, without exception, relatively rare tumors.

1.108 Neurilemmona, Neurofibroma

This is a rare, benign tumor of the nerve sheaths.

Differential diagnosis: not very difficult to differentiate from cysts because it is uneven and rough when palpated; in some cases, it indicates an undetected neurofibromatosis.

Treatment of choice: only excision.

1.109 Recklinghausen's Neurofibrosis

This is a hereditary skin disease.

Differential diagnosis: unmistakable if the clinical picture is pronounced, and more difficult if the tumors or "café au lait" macules occur only singly.

Treatment of choice: no therapy can terminate the disease, but cosmetically and functionally disturbing tumors can be excised.

1.110 Neurofibrosarcoma

This extremely rare tumor is probably generated from the base of a neurofibromatosis.

Treatment of choice: only excision far into the healthy tissue.

1.111 Dysplasias, Hyperplasias, and Fibroses

Differential diagnosis: often difficult to distinguish between tumors such as the keloid and the hypertrophic scar and inflammatory lesions.

1.112 Tylositas Articuli

Treatment of choice: no completely effective treatment is known, and although excision is possible, the tendency to form keloids is strong.

1.113 Palmoplantar Fibrosis (Dupuytren's Contracture)

Treatment of choice: surgical improvement is very promising, but therapy is generally taken over by the hand surgeon.

1.114 Juvenile Palmoplantar Fibrosis

Treatment of choice: besides excision by the hand surgeon, with the danger of recurrence and keloid formation, intralesional corticoid injection presents an alternative.

1.115 Induratio Penis Plastica

Treatment of choice: radiation therapy and intralesional corticosteroid injection are preferable to danger of subsequent impotentia coeundi resulting from surgery.

1.116 Pseudoxanthoma Elasticum

Treatment of choice: surgical correction of individual troublesome lesions possible.

1.117 Cutis Laxa and Cutis Hyperelastica

There is only a slight chance of rehabilitating either of these conditions successfully.

1.118 Inflammatory and Functional Skin Lesions

1.119 Inflammations Originating from Hair Follicles and Sebaceous Glands

1.120 Deep Necrotizing Perifolliculitis

Synonyms: furuncle and carbuncle. These lesions are very common.

Differential diagnosis: generally unproblematic, but on occasion, difficult to differentiate from destroyed follicle cysts, deep trichophytia, or keratoacanthoma.

Treatment of choice: when regression fails to occur, incision. A so-called crucial incision is generally preferable, for a simple incision often conglutinates too quickly. However, the very pronounced scarring that results can be decreased considerably by opening with the rotating, hollow punch [468].

1.121 Dissecting Cellulitis of the Scalp, Periofolliculitis Capitis Abscedens et Suffodiens

Synonyms: acne keloid and folliculitis keloidalis.
Treatment of choice: radical excision combined with antibiotics.

1.122 Dermatitis Perianalis Fistulosa

These lesions, as a rule hardly influenced by antibiotic treatment, lead to extended fistulization.
Treatment of choice: radical opening after which epithelization from the wound edges takes place.

1.123 Pyodermia Fistulans Sinifica

This disorder, belonging to the same category of disorders as dermatitis perianalis fistulosa (Sect. 1.122), is related to acne conglobata and affects the inguinal, perianal, and gluteal areas as well as the axillae.

Differential diagnosis: thought to be hydradenitis suppurativa. Histologically, however, the sweat and apocrine glands are found intact, and the inflammatory lesions are concentrated around dermal sinuses filled with layered horn masses, detritus, and partially destroyed hair follicles. In time, extensive fistulous tracts with constantly recurring inflammations develop.

Treatment of choice: only radical excision stops the recurring suppurations [246] (survey [337]). The functional and cosmetic results achieved after excision and the following epithelization from the wound edges are surprisingly good. We have also witnessed a very good and, most important, very rapid healing following extensive excision into the healthy tissue up to the fascia and subsequent primary repair.

1.124 Acne Conglobata, Acne Abscedens

In serious forms of acne, deeply situated small abscesses and pseudocystic lesions result from blackheads and folliculitis, which frequently have sterile contents, and their removal becomes more difficult the longer they are left intact.

Treatment of choice: Provided the right technique is employed, a simple incision with a lancet causes them to conglutinate quickly: entry with the lancet through the follicle as far as possible, then incision vertically upward toward the opening [306]; rapid conglutination often follows. Subsequently the cystic structure is opened with the rotating hollow punch [249,250]; this results in less scarring than if the inflammation were to continue festering. Supplementing this procedure are the supportive systemic therapy with vitamin A palmitate [233] and the application of external peeling and disinfecting agents such as vitamin A acid or, in some cases, Galuschka's solution (salicylic acid 3.0 g; lactic acid 3.0 g; glycerine 3.0 g; boric acid solution 30.0 g; ethanol 67.00 g). Both have been used with good results. Topical preparations containing corticosteroids should never be used because they generally aggravate the acne rather than combat it.

The development of new cysts and abscesses can be minimized by mechanically eradicating blackheads one of two ways: One method is Unna's blackhead expressor, which is customarily used after applying an antiseptic solution or tincture. The method recorded by Flegel [179] has, however, proved to be even more effective; blackheads are sucked up by a pipette which is placed against the skin and connected to a water jet pump. Scars left by acne can in some cases be corrected by repeated dermabrasion.

1.125 Inflammations Originating in the Sweat Glands, the Odoriferous Glands, and the Mucous Membranes

1.126 Hidradenitis Suppurativa

These are inflammatory lesions which occur primarily in the axillae and groin, perigenitally and perianally.
Differential diagnosis: often difficult

to differentiate from pyodermia fistulans sinifica.
Treatment of choice: early application of a broad-spectrum antibiotic and additional topical disinfectants often causes a rapid abatement. If not cured, a chronically recurring inflammation develops that is frequently accompanied by abscesses, fistulas, and callosities, which can be cured only by radical surgical removal of the affected area [see 316,406].

1.127 Bartholinitis

The recurring inflammations, empyemas, and retention cysts of the Bartholin glands or their excretory ducts are seen less frequently today than before the era of antibiotics.
Differential diagnosis: genuine abscesses are frequently difficult to differentiate.
Treatment of choice: extirpating the unopened cysts under antibiotic protection, preferably during an interval in which there is no inflammation.

1.128 Chronic Inflammations Originating around the Vessels

1.129 Tuberculosis Cutis Luposa

Synonym: lupus vulgaris.
Of all the various forms of skin tuberculosis, lupus is the most likely to require surgical treatment.
Differential diagnosis: some difficulty in differentiating small foci from nevi or histiocytomas in the case of younger patients; from basal cell carcinomas in the case of older patients.
Treatment of choice: therapy is concluded most rapidly by total excision; in any case, thorough physical examination and if necessary, systemic treatment.

1.130 Sarcoidosis (Besnier-Boeck-Schaumann)

The disease is initially diagnosed much more frequently than it actually occurs [147].

Differential diagnosis: occasionally difficulties in differentiating it from, for example, necrobiosis lipoidica, granulomatosis disciformis, and foreign body granulomas.

Treatment of choice: If skin foci are few in number, therapeutic excision and histologic confirmation can often be combined, but general treatment with steroids is nonetheless usually unavoidable since, if correctly diagnosed, it is rare that only the skin is affected [224].

1.131 Cheilitis Granulomatosa (see Sect. 3.044)

1.132 Deep Mycoses and Diseases Due to Actinomyces

Frequently the diagnosis is made only on the basis of histologic and microbiologic examination of excised material.

Treatment of choice: Dealing with a circumscribed infection focus, therapy can often be concluded most quickly and safely by excision of the affected region. Chemotherapy alone is a possible alternative.

1.133 Leishmaniasis

Synonym: oriental sore.

This disease is relatively common among patients from Mediterranean countries and observed in Europe as a vacationer's infection.

Treatment of Choice: total excision and chemotherapy if the foci are few in number.

1.134 Inflammations that Spread to the Skin

In dermatology, the two following lesions are of some importance.

1.135 Dental Skin Fistulas

Differential diagnosis: seldom recognized at the primary stage, they are first treated unsuccessfully when mistaken for perifolliculitis, follicle retention cysts, or acne pustules.

Treatment of choice: No primary dermatosurgical therapy is required because regression usually results after the infected tooth responsible has been extracted. Correction of the scar is occasionally necessary at some later time.

1.136 Tuberculosis Cutis Colliquativa

Synonym: scrofuloderma.

Treatment of choice: combined with chemotherapy or for correction of scar at a later stage.

1.137 Cicatricial Post-inflammatory States and Post-thrombotic Syndrome

1.138 Phimosis

Strictures of the prepuce frequently follow recurring inflammations. During the acute inflammatory stage, local and general antiphlogistic and antibiotic treatment is preferred over surgery, except in the case of the foreskin's retraction (paraphimosis). Then it is necessary to immediately reposition the prepuce; if this cannot be done, dorsal incision is imperative.

Treatment of choice: circumcision after the inflammatory symptoms have disappeared.

1.139 Superficial Thrombophlebitis

This lesion is only briefly touched upon here because of its relation to the following diagnoses (1.140–1.145).

Treatment of choice: in particular the procedure published by Sigg [459], consisting of a longitudinal incision approximately ¾ in. (2 cm) into the palpably thrombosed vessel. After the thrombus is manually expressed, a compression dressing is applied, which promotes very rapid disappearance of the symptoms, in contrast to conservative therapy which proves rather ineffective.

1.140 Varicosis in Chronic Venous Insufficiency

At present time, surgical therapy for varicosis is performed mainly by vascular surgeons, although the dermatologist usually recommends the therapy. Examination suffices to show if the great or the lesser saphenous vein is affected. Only genuine varices are not very common. If the valves are functioning, there is no evidence of skin disease.

On the other hand, postthrombotic conditions frequently occur even when the anamnesis is inconclusive. Examination for this condition involves the following: First, the functioning of the valves is checked according to procedures by Schwartz and Trendelenburg I; the sufficiency of the femoral veins and the communicating veins, according to methods of Perthes, Trendelenburg II, Linton, and Mehorner-Ochsner; and the location of the communicating veins is checked ac-

cording to the method of Albanese [cf. 197,268] and marked when it is determined.

If necessary phlebography can be used for comparison purposes in order to locate the course of the communicating veins and of occlusions of the deep veins. The more exact these clinical tests are, the more valuable they are.

Treatment of choice: Depending on the specifics of the individual case, sclerosing therapy or surgical removal is recommended. If occlusions of the deep veins are found, treatment should not exclude sclerosing of superficial vascular components which clearly allow backflow [459]. Pronounced insufficiency of the great saphenous vein calls for the Keller-Babcock operation with its more recent modifications [247]. Large individual varix conglomerates with slight stasis can also be marked externally, doubly ligated, and then surgically removed through small incisions. Another procedure is used for especially insufficient communicating veins. After external marking, they are located by small skin incisions, followed into the deep layers, and after the fascia is split, ligated with nonresorbent suture material.

Sclerosing therapy is preferred when dealing with all smaller peripheral varices, regardless of their total extent, because of its positive results and its repeatability. As a complement to both therapies, correctly applied elastic bandages are just as much a prerequisite for success in operative measures as they are in injection therapy.

1.141 Small Varicose Dilatations of Cutaneous Veins

Treatment of choice: sclerosing therapy is recommended for these lesions, which are often cosmetically detracting [459]. However, the treatment can be rather difficult, especially when handling very small veins; since they are difficult to puncture and compress, discharges and pigmentations often result.

An alternative is the use of an electric needle, which neatly scleroses these fine vein components (as well as spider nevi or teleangiectasias in connection with corticoid skin injuries or rosacea). In this procedure—anesthesia rarely proving necessary—a fine electric needle is injected at low current in close proximity to the vein, the foot pedal being pressed for only a split second at a time. The vein will pale, but the surrounding area should not turn whitish in color. After a few sessions, the varicoses disappear without leaving any scars. Follow-up treatment consists in applying a thin layer of antiphlogistic cream on the first day.

1.142 Pachydermia Vegetans and Papillomatosis Cutis

The treatment of basic lymphatic and venous outflow disturbances is essential for the success of any therapy (see below). If necessary, the fibrotic skin area is excised as well and the wound repaired by a split-thickness graft.

1.143 Dermatopathy of the Leg

This is a minor sclerosis of the skin on the calves.

Treatment of choice: After several years of successful therapy for blood and lymph outflow disturbances, it disappears and does not of itself require surgery. However, because of the ulcers arising from poor blood supply to the tissue, incision or circumcision must frequently be performed.

1.144 Elephantiasis Nostras

This chronic lymphedema, occurring particularly in the lower extremities and the genital area, results from chronic streptococci infections, frequently developing in skin lesions due to foot mycoses.

Treatment of choice: Surgery often presents the only chance for improvement, presupposing, of course, good equipment, access to a hospital, and capable staff. Since the more advanced procedures of integumentectomy or displacement of fascia lata strips are not very common, the Handley-Zieman technique [358] is recommended. In this procedure, monofile plastic threads are implanted so as to extend in a proximal direction far into an area where outflow conditions are intact.

1.145 Leg Ulcer

Variant: "ulcus cruris venosum."

This disease is related to postthrombophlebitic chronic venous insufficiency. The occlusion of the femoral veins is diagnostically verified by examining [117] the extent and location of the underlying disorder (for example, insufficiency of the great or lesser saphenous veins or of communicating veins).

Treatment of choice: depending on the case specifics, either surgery [174,197,247] or sclerosing [165,459, 574] of the main venous disorder is chosen. Then the ulcer is repaired after being debrided with conservative therapy or surgically freshened using Thiersch's grafts or Reverdin's pinch grafts [392] and a split-thickness graft [155]. The split-thickness graft has the advantage of being easily repeated several times if it does not take the first time. The same holds true for the "skin cultivation'' procedure [146], in which epidermis scrapings from the thigh are deposited in the ulcer, which is kept moist with a cultivating solution. The advantages of this treatment are that there is no scar left at the donor site and there should be few preconditions on the state of the ulcer.

1.146 Arteriosclerotic and Diabetic Gangrene of the Leg

The dermatologist's usually conservative therapy is combined with the internist's treatment of the primary disorder. If, however, the defect cannot be healed, the last possibility is amputation.

1.147 Lesions Due to Foreign Bodies and Trauma

1.148 Foreign Body Granuloma

Most commonly occurring on the face and hands, this is often clinically mistaken for a keloid.
Treatment of choice: excision in toto.

1.149 Tattoos and Other Corial Foreign Body Intrusions

Treatment of choice: single-step or total excision performed in several sessions, chemical cauterization, curettage, or dermabrasion [104,145, 295,307]. However, due to the deeply situated pigments in the corium, excision is very frequently the only procedure which completely and finally eradicates the lesions with tolerable scarring.

1.150 Keloid. (cf. Sect. 1.068)

1.151 Traumatic Epithelial Cysts (cf. Sect. 1.019)

1.152 Chondrodermatitis Nodularis Chronica Helicis Winkler

This common reactive, inflammatory lesion occurs on the upper edge of the auricle, predominantly among men over 40 years of age.
Differential diagnosis: solar keratosis or carcinoma.
Treatment of choice: the only treatment promising success is excision into the healthy tissue.

1.153 Callosities, Tyloma

Synonyms: tylosities and callus.
This extension of connective tissue (Sect. 1.119) generally lies below the thickened stratum coreum on skin areas under mechanical strain. Callosities not normally excised require suitable topical treatment, for the affected skin shows a tendency to fissure formation and high infection. However, an exception to this are the recurring inflammatory callosities on the balls of the big toes, found primarily in female diabetics and recently differentiated by Illig as a separate syndrome. The deep, extensive fistulas often lie hidden underneath and are usually cured only by extensive surgery.

1.154 Burns and Scalding

Patients with extensive, serious burns are generally referred to special burn centers, but the dermatologist usually deals with circumscribed first- and second-degree burns and small areas of third-degree burn foci, especially in connection with household accidents.

Treatment of choice: after initially cooling the burn in cold water at the scene of or directly following the accident, further treatment is, for the most part, conservative. Shock therapy, needed under certain circumstances, open wound treatment, or salve dressing technique will not be reviewed here. Provisional foreign skin transplantation is unnecessary for most small burn areas, and extirpation of destroyed tissue components need not be as substantial as for serious burns. Of prime importance, however, is the plastic repair of those components suffering third-degree burns and not epithelizing from the skin appendages. Full-thickness skin grafts should be employed over joints when possible because of the tendency of split-thickness grafts to shrink.

1.155 Chemical Burns

Treatment of choice: after extensive rinsing under running water (usually available at the scene of the accident), buffers of finely dispersed protein (evaporated milk) are recommended in some instances.

Warning: the widespread "treatment" of applying acid cauteries with diluted alkali or alkali with diluted acid only causes further injury. If during conservative treatment certain sites do not reepithelize from the skin appendages due to deep destruction, then plastic repair is necessary.

1.156 Wounds

Almost every physician is constantly confronted with the treatment of various small skin injuries. Before treatment, it is necessary to determine whether foreign bodies have entered the wound, especially in the case of automobile accidents. It is also important to consider the cosmetic and functional results and possible plastic repair before simply suturing the wound.

1.157 Suture Dehiscence

The removal of sutures for cosmetic reasons soon after minor operations entails a certain risk of suture dehiscence due to mechanical strain. To obviate this risk, suture tape is applied while the sutures are being pulled. If the suture gaps, the wound can generally be closed by using only this type of suture dressing, for tension is now far slighter than at the time of the first treatment. The dressing remains in situ for a week. If the wound edges cannot easily be adapted by this means, a new suture of the wound is made immediately without any risk. However, it is a more serious matter if the dehiscence cannot be treated promptly, for then the whole wound must be excised and resutured. Yet even in this case today, results superior to secondary healing are achieved.

1.158 Functional and Cosmetic Disorders

1.159 Axillary Hyperhidrosis

Treatment of choice: since conservative treatment brings no results, X-ray therapy, still widely practiced, is considered unacceptable [38]; the only effective measure is excision [see 258,399,407]. Using Minor's sweat test if necessary, the dimension and form of the area in question are determined and then excised in a longitudinal, or more often, transversely shaped ellipse, which is closed with interrupted sutures.

1.160 Cosmetic Surgery

Disorders such as blepharochalasis, rehabilitation of disturbing forehead wrinkles, baggy cheeks, double chin, pendulous abdomen, etc., generally belong to the realm of cosmetic surgery; only under circumstances requiring certain medical treatment do they become the object of dermatosurgery [18]. The basic techniques for treating such disorders are presented according to their location. For example, operations for baldness, which sometimes result in a scarred bald spot years later, will be discussed briefly under surgical techniques for the scalp area.

1.161 Lesions of the Nails

Two diseases of the nails often justify minor operations in dermatology: onychomyoses and ingrown toenail.

1.162 Onychomycoses

Treatment of choice: first the conservative therapy for removing nail plate and debris; this is the Araviskij method of applying daily equal parts of potassium-iodide and lanolin in powder form under a plastic film (such as Saran Wrap), possibly following curettage or else using cream containing antimycotics under plastic film. If unsuccessful, the only course remaining is nail extraction under conduction anesthesia with systemic antimycotic treatment as a follow-up. An injection of hyaluronidase under the nail facilitates removal, although the nail bed usually has to be curetted afterward. The recurrence rate following use of systemic griseofulvin therapy is high, even when complementing extraction. Most salves and tinctures are not alternatives to extraction, because they do not penetrate the nail. Only in extreme cases and under clinical conditions (for example, if disturbances in the arterial blood supply make extraction hazardous) can the use of nail removal solution containing strontium sulfide pulp be condoned.

1.163 Ingrown Toenail

Treatment of choice: Conservative treatment as well as the frequent practice of stuffing gauze strips under nail corners is not effective, and extraction of only the nail almost always leads to recurrences. However, the Emmet surgical procedure [158] makes recurrence unlikely, while at the same time achieving a fine cosmetic result. After a fairly wide lateral nail and nail bed component are excised, epithelization occurs from the edges.

2. Basic Principles of Dermatosurgery: Survey of Surgical Techniques*

2.001 Requirements and Considerations

The decision whether to perform surgery depends on the general condition of the patient [242,243,396]. If, for example, there are substantial internal contraindications, another method of treatment will be preferred or, in the case of cosmetic corrections [405], treatment will be refused [244]. On the other hand, the after effects of other therapeutic measures, e.g., especially radiation [266,455,496], are frequently a reason for operating. Late radiation injuries [radiation combination injuries, cf. 287,379] are treated relatively frequently by the dermatologist [480]. Therapy for these injuries is always surgical [288,355,401,572], especially if cancer is suspected [26,178,336,374, 415]. Conservative local therapy ensures that the area for surgery [500,509] is properly prepared. Minor operations are performed under local anesthesia. If more extensive plastic surgery is necessary, a physical examination must ascertain whether the patient is healthy enough for full anesthesia and an operation. The anesthesiologist is consulted on whether to use local or gen-

eral anesthesia. In addition to its aesthetic improvements, surgical treatment of tumors is recommended [125,134] for the following:

1. To prevent malignant neogeneses in the case of skin lesions, e.g., solar keratosis, leukoplakia, lentigo maligna, lupus vulgaris, and late radiation injury [170,323,368,424].

2. In the presence of neoplasms near bones or cartilage (nasal tip, auricle, larynx, temple regions, scalp, hands, feet, phalanges, etc.) to obviate the danger of cartilage or bone necrosis resulting from x-ray therapy applied to the neoplasms [19,93,344]. Additionally, the sluggish reaction of the veins in the temporal and parietal region [325,326], for example, negatively influences radiation treatment in this area [27], and when there are neogeneses on the scalp, there is the frequently unavoidable danger of radiogenic epilation.

3. For special tumors such as morphea-like basal cell carcinoma or highly differentiated squamous cell carcinoma, which respond only slightly to radiation [159,160]. As a general rule, any suspicious lesion which has not responded after 1–2 months of conservative treatment should be excised [107,332] and examined histologically [214]. In this manner a possible neo-

---

*[See 24,189,406].

plasm is verified, its continued growth prevented, and the danger of recurrence reduced [32,349].

In the case of benign neogeneses and nontumorous lesions, excision just within the healthy tissue is sufficient.

However, with malignant neogeneses and especially with neoplasms tending to local recurrence [169], an adequate safety margin must be maintained on the sides as well as in the depth of the tissue layers [284,370,448] so as to prevent a recurrence of the neoplasm in the same area [88,191,350]. If there is any difficulty in ascertaining the extent of the excision macroscopically, an intraoperative frozen section of the margins of resection must be performed; an incomplete excision of a malignant tumor demands immediate resection far into the healthy tissue [162].

In basal cell carcinomas, nodular forms [472] require a safety margin of only a few millimeters (1/16 in.); those belonging to ulcus rodens or ulcus terebrans, a wider margin; and morphea-like basal cell carcinomas, an extensive excision monitored with a frozen section [cf. 309]. When dealing with a well-differentiated squamous cell carcinoma, however, a safety margin of 1–2 cm (½–¾ in.) is desirable; for malignant melanoma, the safety margin must be at least 5 cm (2 in.) [69,89, 211,333] from the clinically visible edge of the tumor. Optimally every tumor patient should be followed for a number of years following surgery [142,161,162] to discover recurrence or lymph node metastases as early as possible.

Plastic repair of the defect is preferred to a primary suture with an excision that is too large [198,268,383], especially in regions of the body where there is relatively little surrounding skin available for closing the wound (head and extremities, for instance, [cf. 81]). Obviously the operation must be as radical as possible if dealing with malignant neogeneses [7,140,380], but removing a tumor in toto is, nevertheless, not enough. An attempt should always be made to achieve aesthetically pleasing surgical results [134,257].

This can be done by making the incision line so that the suture rests in one of the relaxed skin tension lines (Fig. 1). This requirement is not always possible, for skin tension lines do not always correspond to skin fissure lines [310], but it is especially feasible if the wound is closed by a primary suture or "Dehnungsplastik" (Sect. 2.18).

When dealing with local flaps, transposition or advancement flaps, for instance, care must be taken to situate the operation scars in preformed creases and to avoid, when possible, sensitive structures such as the mimic musculature and the larger vessels and nerves (Fig. 2a–c).

Free autologous skin transplants used in repairing surgical defects should be taken from donor sites with approximately the same structure [43]. Skin flaps from the upper eyelid and the retroauricular and supraclavicular regions are especially well suited for transplantation in the nasal and cheek regions. Skin replacement on the forehead can be made from the inner side of the upper arm.

2.002 Surgical Instruments

The choice of correct surgical instruments [cf. 397] frequently determines the course of healing and the aesthetic result. Coarse forceps, large needles,

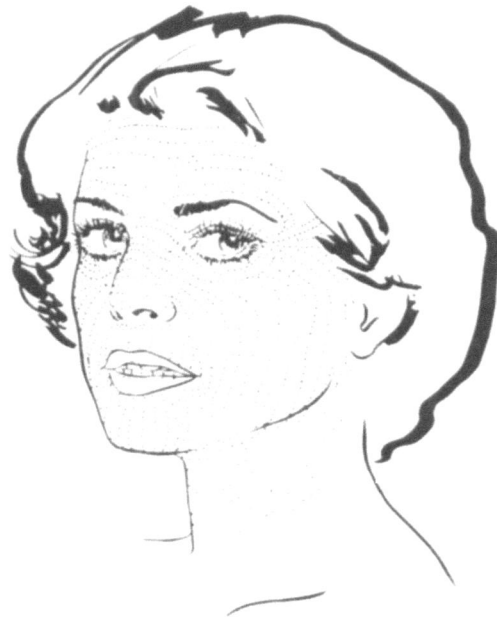

Fig. 1. *"Relaxed skin tension lines."*

unwieldy needle holders and scissors traumatize the wound edges, causing microthrombi and superficial necroses which lead to a wide scar. Needle holders with the smallest grips possible must be used with small roundbodied needles to prevent the needles' bending or breaking off in the tissue. Atraumatic suture material is preferred, especially in such cases where the resulting scars will not be hidden by clothing (face and hands) and when the operation is primarily for aesthetic reasons.

2.003 Pre- and Postoperative Care

With general anesthesias, the patient must eat and drink nothing for at least 6 hours prior to the operation. To prevent law suits in the case of an anesthesia accident, he must be explicitly warned that failure to comply with the requirement invites possible asphyxiation. Even operations under local anesthesia should follow this rule when possible, in order to reduce the risk of an emergency intubation if the patient goes into shock [451].

In preparing nonambulatory adult patients for operation, it is helpful to administer a sedative the evening before the operation; children receive proportionately smaller doses.

If the operation is performed under local anesthesia, the patient should receive an ampule of Vesprin or 2 ml Innovar [114] and in every case 0.25–0.6 mg atropine as vagolyticum half an hour before the operation. The patient is injected with this medication in the ward, at which time he is cautioned not to leave his bed again because of the danger of collapsing. Patients are

FACIAL NERVES

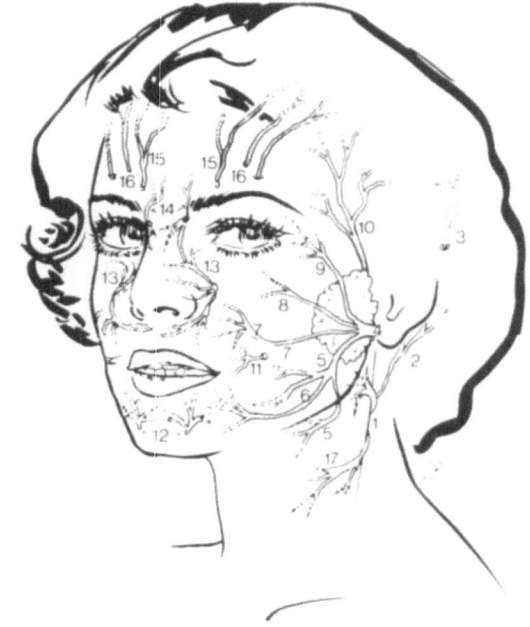

 1 Great auricular n.
 2 Smaller occipital n.
 3 Greater occipital n.
 4 Facial n.
 5 Cervical branch
 6 Marginal mandibular branch
 7 Buccal branch
 8 Zygomatic branch
 9 Temporal branch
10 Auriculotemporal n.
11 Buccal n.
12 R. & L. Mental n.
13 Infraorbital n.
14 Supra & Infratrochlear n.
15 Supraorbital n. (medial)
16 Supraorbital n. (lateral)
17 Cervical transverse n.

a

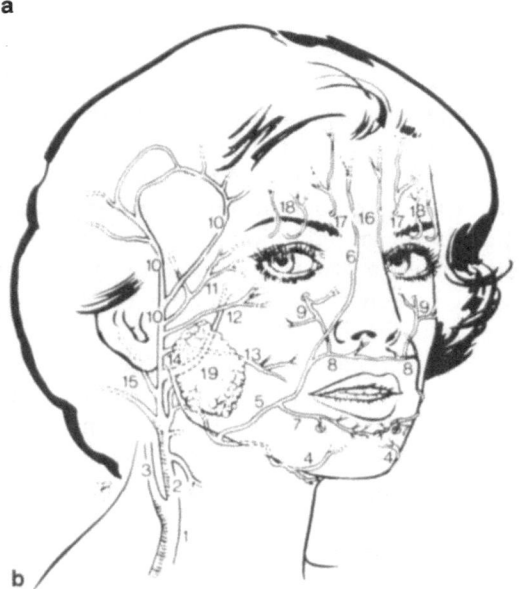

b

FACIAL ARTERIES

 1 Common carotid a.
 2 External carotid a.
 3 Internal carotid a.
 4 Submental a.
 5 Facial a.
 6 Augular a.
 7 Inferior labial a.
 8 Superior a.
 9 Infraorbital a.
10 Superficial temporal a.
   (Frontal and parietal branches)
11 Zygomaticoorbital a.
12 Medial temporal a.
13 Transverse facial a.
14 Maxillary a.
15 Occipital a.
16 Supratrochlear a. (medial)
17 Supratrochlear a. (lateral)
18 Supraorbital a.
19 Parotid gland

Fig. 2. a–c *Anatomic features of most important facial structures* to be considered during facial surgery. Special attention must be paid to: the forehead: the frontal a. and n.; the nose and the canthus: the lacrymal duct, the angular a. and v.; the nasolabial region: the facial a. and v. and the zygomatic m.; the auricular region: frontal and temporal branches of the superficial temporal a., the retroauricular a. and the facial nerve. If one considers the structure of the oral musculature, the course of the branches of the facial nerve, as well as the maxillary, labila, facial, and mandibular arteries, the advantage of the vermillionectomy over triangular excisions becomes clear.

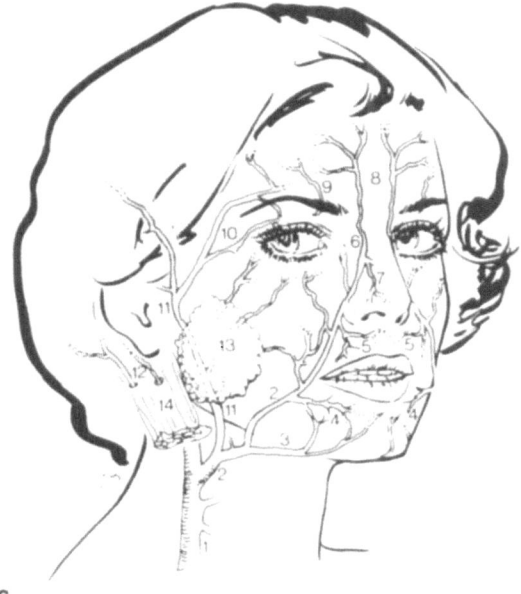

FACIAL VEINS

1 Internal jugular v.
2 Facial v.
3 Submental v.
4 Inferior labial v.
5 Superior labial v.
6 Augular v.
7 External nasal v.
8 Supratrochlear v.
9 Supraorbital v.
10 Superficial temporalis v.
11 Retromandibular v.
12 Retroauricular v.
13 Parotid gland
14 Sternocleidomastoid muscle

c

brought into the operating room lying down and transferred there from their bed to the operating table. In the case of ambulatory patients, premedication is not necessary before local anesthesia. After the hospitalized patients receive their premedication, the area to be operated on is adequately shaved.

Despite low excitation during modern administration of anesthesia, it is recommended that patients be secured to the operating table, especially children and infants, because of the danger that patients roll over to the side and fall off the operating table on awaking from the anesthesia. A softly padded strap fastened over the abdomen and hips prevents such accidents.

Another danger is superextension. When positioning the patient, care must be taken not to superextend and to avoid nerve lesions. Since branches of the brachial plexus are especially prone to becoming strained and slightly paralyzed due to incorrect positioning of the body, the arm should neither be rotated much outwardly nor drawn more than 90 degrees away from the body. After full relaxation, no part of the body must be allowed to extend over a metal edge of the table.

During operations on the head, the cervical spinal column may not be superextended, for older patients are likely to have arthritic lesions in this area. Indeed, cervical spine fractures have resulted in some cases from poor positioning [194]. Finally, special caution must be observed when changing the position of anesthetized patients since protective reflexes and reflectory muscle tension are absent.

The area to be operated on is cleaned preoperatively with disinfecting solutions. Any residue of these substances, especially around body orifices (female genitals, auricular canal), must be removed promptly because of the danger of toxic reactions. If the disinfectant can possibly come into contact with the eyelids or the conjunctival sac, a protective ointment must be applied to this area beforehand. Taping the lid fissure with a narrow nonirritating bandage also helps avoid painful and long-lasting conjunctivitis [194]. When electrocautery is used, the grounding electrode must lie as flatly on the skin as possible. To prevent burns on the anesthetized patient, the metal parts of the connection pieces must not touch the patient's skin.

An antimicrobial powder is applied after closure of the wound by primary suture or Dehnungsplastik. The wound is then covered by a compress fastened with a minimally irritating tape. The powder should not contain talcum because of the danger of foreign body granulomas ("talcum granuloma") or keloids. For skin grafts or flaps, fatty tulle is the preferred wound covering because it prevents a stasis of wound secretion and the adherence of the wound dressing that is fixed over the operation area with semielastic gauze bandages. When dealing with free skin transplants in the extremities, it is advisable to immobilize the patient, including the joints nearest the transplant, for 8–10 days by means of a plaster cast.

An optimal bandaging technique can effectively help prevent transplant necroses and secondary wound healing. Fully anesthetized patients must be watched over after surgery until they are again completely conscious.

In order to minimize the chances of a postoperative edema, antiphlogistic drugs may be prescribed as a prophylactic measure. In view of the asepsis of the skin surface, which is only partially achievable, the additional administration of broad spectrum antibiotics may be effective in more extensive surgical procedures. In plastic operations resulting in larger wound areas, continuous suction by means of plastic tubing is used to prevent the formation of hematomas and seromas [24,189].

2.004 Anesthesia Procedures

Adequate anesthesia is prerequisite to the successful performance and conclusion of an operation [11]. The extent of the planned operation permitting, local anesthesia is usually preferred; more extensive operations, which would require too great a quantity of local anesthetics, necessitate general anesthesia or, in the area of the extremities, lumbar or plexus anesthesia. The anesthesiologist is consulted on this procedure.

One advantage of local anesthesia is that the patient is conscious during the operation. This is of great significance in operations in critical areas (facial nerves, nerves of the extremities) since only the conscious patient can take an active role in monitoring his functions. However, disadvantage lies in the fact that an injection of local anesthesia creates an edema of the wound edges, making exact adaption of the wound margin difficult. Similarly, in complicated operations in the facial area, e.g., in plastic lip surgery, the necessary distortion of soft parts from infiltrated local anesthetic impedes adjustment of differences and, in some instances, even endangers the final result [153]. In major operations on children and infants, general anesthesia and possibly ketamine analgesia are necessary.

The disadvantages of general anesthesia in contrast to local anesthesia are the greater frequency of hermorrhaging in the operated area and the increased danger to heart and blood circulation. Today, however, a skillful anesthesiologist can considerably minimize these risks [441].

2.005 Local Anesthesia (for techniques, cf. [11,330])

Every physician should know the basic principles of intubation, extrathoracular heart massage, and phlebotomy. The operating room should be equipped with the means for reanimation and therapy in case of shock, i.e., endotracheal spatula, tube, and oxygen equipment. Epinephrine, water-soluble corticoids, and plasma expanders should always be at hand.

2.006 Local Anesthetics

Local anesthetics such as lidocaine and mepivacaine are preferred since, contrary to earlier statements [100], benzocaine or procaine preparations pose a greater risk of allergic complications. The amount should not exceed 30–40 ml of 1% solution per session. After ½ h an additional 5 cc can be injected, if necessary. Adding epinephrine to the anesthetic (up to 1: 200,000) causes a temporary constriction of the blood vessels, thus reducing intraoperative hemorrhaging and improving visibility in the region being operated on. However, these advantages must be disregarded in the distal parts of the extremities since the vasoconstriction caused by the adrenalin can lead to necroses there.

Warning: "surface anesthesia" with ethyl-chloride spray, still customary today in some places, must not be used because of its dubious effectiveness, the toxicity of the agent, and the danger of explosion.

2.007 Marginal Wall Anesthesia

It is not advisable to inject the anesthetic directly into the region of operation, for in the case of malignant tumors the spreading of tumor cells may result. Likewise, the fine structure of the excised tissue may be impaired by an edema caused by direct injection. It is recommended that the anesthetic be administered in two injections (for larger neoplasms, several) made in a fan shape around the focus. By moving the needle forward, the danger of intravascular injection can be avoided to a large extent.

2.008 Conduction Anesthesia

The local anesthetic is injected proximally to the operation field into the area of the supplying sensory nerves (for survey see [324]). This method is used for operations on toes and fingers, as well as on the male genitalia. On the phalanges the injection is made medially and laterally from the proximal joint (cf. Fig. 3). When the anesthesia is correctly placed, the distal phalanx is anesthetized within 5–10 min.

The same procedure applies to the penis. The injection is given dorsally on both sides of the penis root in the area of the dorsal nerve. From the injection site the needle is pushed forward extrafascially under the loose pliable skin and the anesthetic is administered over the entire circumference. The genitofemoral nerve can also be anesthetized

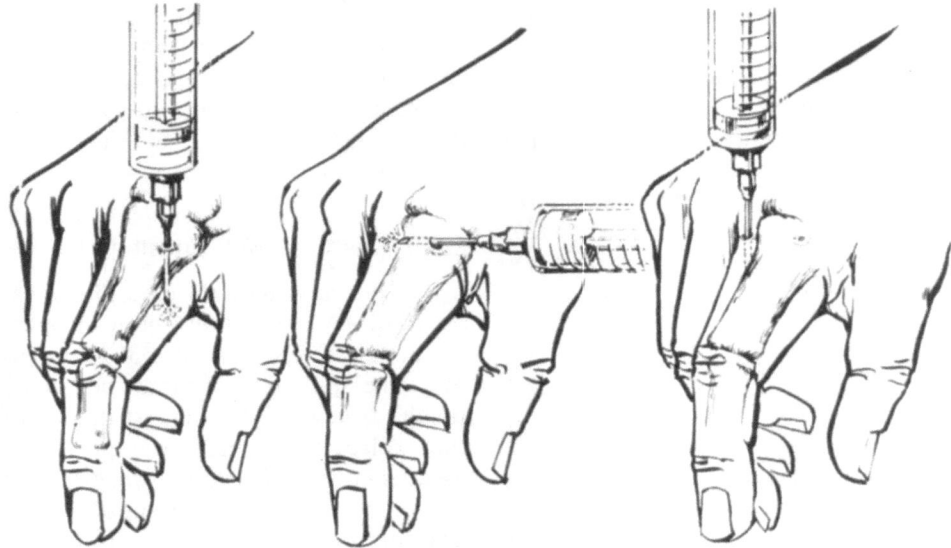

Fig. 3. *Conduction anesthesia* in the area of the proximal finger joint.

by injecting a depot in the region of the inguinal canal. When treating condylomas in the area of the corona of the glans penis and the frenulum or when performing circumcision, additional infiltration of the corona and the frenulum is recommended.

Warning. Do not add epinephrine to the anesthetic for use on the phalanges and penis (end arteries!).

2.009 Special Regional Anesthesia Procedures

As a rule, these special procedures should be carried out by the anesthesiologist. They include complete anesthetization of the hand (not a simple technique), e.g., injection of local anesthetic in the region of the wrist bone; the equally difficult foot blockade by injection of a local anesthetic in the area of the median and lateral ankle bone; the plexus blockade by injection in the brachial plexus (*Warning:* avoid

pneumothorax); epidural anesthesia by injection between the spinal apophyses into the extradural area near the yellow ligament; spinal anesthesia by injection into the subarachnoid area surrounding the spinal cord; and sacral anesthesia by injection into the extradural area of the sacral canal.

2.010 General Anesthesia

In major operations in the field of dermatosurgery, intubation anesthesia is preferred to local anesthesia. In facial surgery, intubation from the upper lip should be made orotracheally and in operations on the lower lip, nasotracheally [365]. Halothane, used frequently in inhalation anesthesia, does not prevent skin transplants from conglutinating [376]. However, because intubation anesthesia requires extensive equipment and personnel and necessitates postoperative care, such operations are generally limited to the hospital.

2.011 Incisions and Suture Techniques

It is important for the cosmetic aspect of a surgical scar that the incision is made as vertically as possible to the surface of the skin. This considerably facilitates an exact adaption of the wound edges. Bleeding subcutaneous vessels, especially in the facial region, should be individually pinched and ligated with atraumatic catgut (3–0 to 5–0) or cauterized with electrocautery. Subcutaneous sutures are made only if absolutely necessary, and then as few as possible using thin catgut, for a disrupted resorption occasionally leads to foreign body granulomas.

2.012 Interrupted Sutures

To reduce foreign body irritation these should be knotted as finely as possible with monofile polyester or silk thread, for these materials are especially nonirritating to tissue. The advantages of polyester sutures are its tensile strength and easy manipulation.

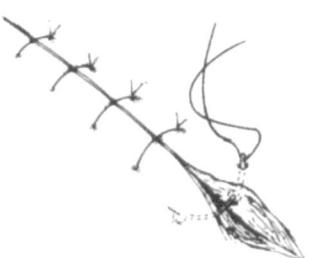

If layered with Teflon and silicone, its serrate effect and a cutting of the skin are minimized. In view of these qualities, silk is inferior to the modern synthetic suture material; however, it allows the placement of exact knots without constricting the tissue [195]. On visible sites, needle insertion and

removal should not take place with more than a 1–2 mm margin from the wound edge. It is not necessary to pull wound edges together by sutures; on the contrary, it is better to bring them together gently with several fine sutures [100]. On the face, atraumatic suture material is used, as a rule No. 5–0 or even 6–0 on eyelids and lips.

2.013 Mattress Sutures

They are performed when necessary as U sutures (strength of the suture material: face, 4–0; scalp and trunk, 3–0 to 1–0).

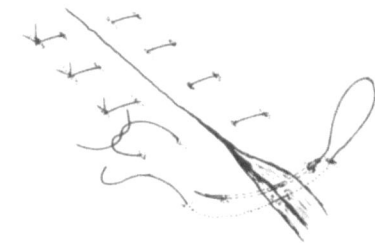

2.014 Continuous Intradermic Suture

Based on our experience, the cosmetic results of this technique (for survey see [269]) are not considerably superior to those of the interrupted suture, for the threads occasionally break, especially in the case of larger wounds. Moreover, if thread remnants are left in the tissue, foreign body granulomas and keloids may result [471].

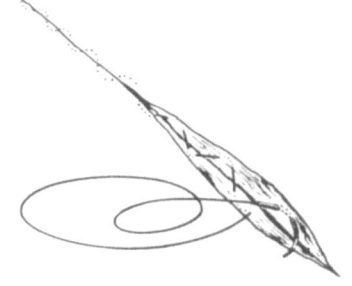

Therefore this suture technique is used by us only rarely.

2.015 Removal of Sutures

An early removal of suture usually avoids cutting by sutures and so-called suture suppurations, thus improving the cosmetic result. Facial sutures should be removed 3 or 4 days after the operation, or 7 or 8 days at the latest; on the trunk and in the region of the extremities, 7 or 8 days later, if the healing process is without complications; and in an exceptional case, even later (mattress sutures, extreme wound tension).

2.016 Surgical Techniques

2.017 Skin Biopsy

This operation [51] is especially important in dermatology, because it is indispensable for making a diagnosis and verifying large numbers of dermatoses (cf. also [68,428]) and can also be used to plan the operation, especially if it contributes to ruling out a malignant neogenesis. Thus, the patient is spared more extensive plastic surgery if a larger safety margin from the tumor edge is not required. It is, however, impossible to determine the extent of a tumor's spread and depth by biopsy alone [32,285,393] since frequently only a part of the tumor is visible on the surface of the skin [283]. Generally, skin biopsies are employed in cases where malignant and semimalignant neogeneses of the epidermis and the connective tissue are suspected; however, radical excision is preferred if it is not much more extensive than the biopsy, which only serves as a verification of the diagnosis before radiation therapy (cf. also [147,221]). If malignant melanoma is suspected, a biopsy should not be performed because of the danger of spreading tumor cells into the bloodstream. Removal of the tissue must be performed far enough to the side and into the deep layers to permit a histologic diagnosis.

In principle, two techniques of diagnostic skin biopsy are possible:

1. Elliptical excision using the scalpel and subsequent wound closure with one or two interrupted sutures.

2. Tissue removal with the punch (diameter: 1–10 mm, tissue depth: 5–8 mm). In order to avoid cauterizing the excision edge, it is absolutely necessary to guide high speed rotating punches quickly through the skin [465]. The tissue cylinder is lifted with an atraumatic forceps and is cut with scissors where it connects to the subcutis. The wound is then closed with one or two interrupted sutures. Punch wounds should not be allowed to heal secondarily without suturing, because cosmetically unfavorable scarring would result. The scar from a large punch wound, closed by suture, is less noticeable than that from an unsutured 2-mm punch, but the punch technique alone is not a "scarless" surgical procedure [249] and it does not meet today's cosmetic standards. This method should not be used if the subcutis is only minimally developed and if there is a danger of injuring deeper tissue layers, e.g., tentous periostem.

2.018 Elliptical Excision with Primary Wound Closure

Following elliptical excision of the focus, the wound is closed by adaption of the edges with an interrupted or con-

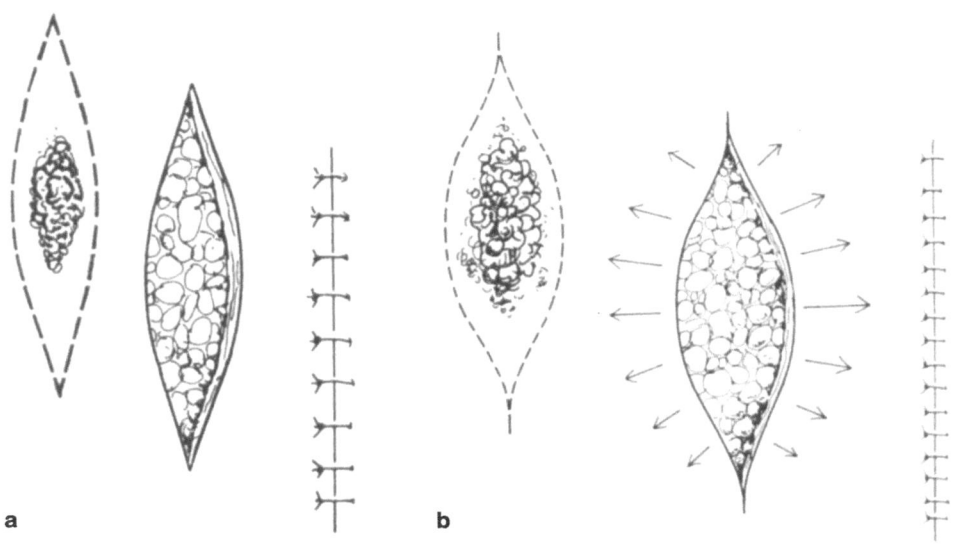

Fig. 4. a, *Elliptical excision with primary wound closure.* **b,** *"Dehnungsplastik"* for a large elliptical wound. The wound is closed by primary suture after undermining the surrounding skin areas.

tinuous intradermic suture. To achieve better wound edge adaption it may be necessary to make some subcutaneous catgut sutures (cf. Fig. 4a). The ovular excision frequently recommended is scarcely possible if the incision is made in a straight vertical line, and moreover, it leads to protrusions at both ends.

2.019 "Dehnungsplastik" (Friederich [19])

If there are large elliptically shaped surgical defects, the surrounding skin areas are undermined subcutaneously by means of dissecting scissors [cf. also 126,127]. Using this technique, the skin stretches and the primary closure of the wound, previously impossible, is achieved. The placement of a few sub-cutaneous sutures improves wound edge adaption and facilitates a closure (either interrupted or continuous intradermic) that is free of tension later (cf. Fig. 4b).

If excision with primary suture even after "Dehnungsplastik" no longer suffices to repair the defect, more extensive plastic surgical methods must be applied [41,46,58,108,136,155,166,240, 282,286,367,446,449,461]. These are of particular importance in skin tumor surgery when an operation must be performed with an adequately large safety margin. When dealing with a tumor recurrence, a second operation is much more extensive and there is less chance of a permanent cure [343]. The methods used in executing regional flaps near the wound and those in other parts of the body are different in principle.

2.020 Regional Flaps

The vascular supply of the flap must be considered when planning the operation to avoid unnecessary transplant necroses [437].

2.021 Z-Flap Technique

By interchanging two triangular skin flaps [478], tissue shrinkage is successfully avoided and the tension corrected within a linear scar. Angles of approximately 60° are necessary in plotting the "Z." This method is recommended particularly for the extremities, nose, eyelids, lips, and neck [282] (Fig. 5a).

Multiple Z flaps are the therapy of choice for correcting scars caused by accidents [30,31,305]. Skin tension lines should be observed in order to minimize visible scarring [72] (cf. Fig. 5b).

2.022 VY-Flap Technique

According to this technique, a V-shaped incision is made first, then the peritomized skin region is undermined or freely prepared, and finally the "V" is stretched; a "Y" suture results and thus the tissue is extended. This technique (cf. Fig. 6) is as suitable as the Z-flap for correcting skin tension contractions as well as minor tissue loss.

Preferred region of application: nose, eyelids, lips, and neck [24,400].

A bipedicled VY-flap (VYS-plasty, according to Argamaso) closes round-shaped to ovular-shaped tissue defects and splits up long linear scars, which are not aesthetically satisfying.

2.023 Advancement Flap Technique

According to the information of von Burow [49], the focus is excised in the shape of a triangle, the short side of the triangle then extended laterally, cranially, or caudally, and a Burow triangle excised on the contralateral side. After undermining the skin area lying between the primary surgical wound and the Burow triangle, it is advanced and the operation defect closed free of tension (cf. Fig. 7).

Preferred region of application: head and trunk.

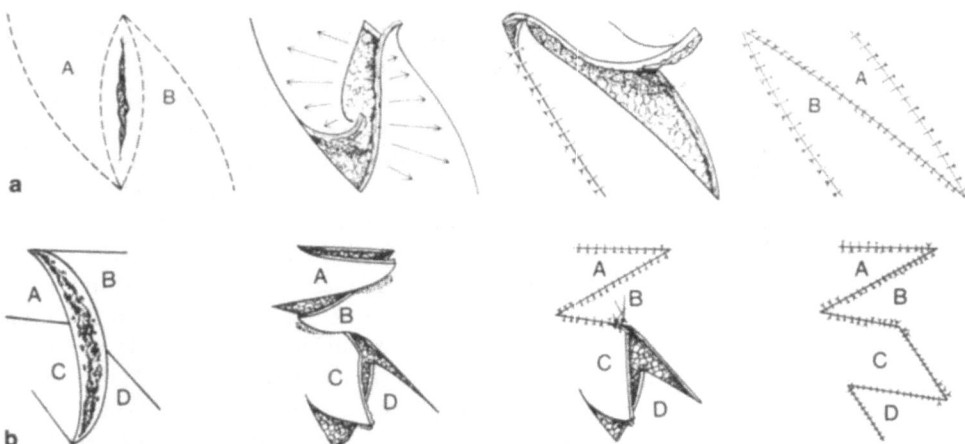

Fig. 5. a, *Z-flap technique.* **b,** *Multiple Z-flaps technique* in correcting unattractive facial scars.

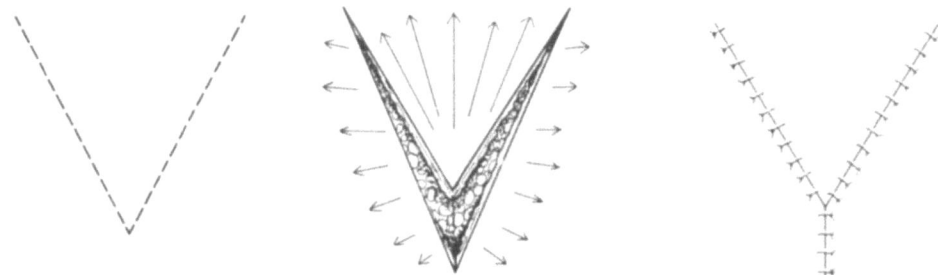

Fig. 6. *VY-flap technique.* After making a "V"-shaped incision and undermining, the "V" is extended longitudinally. The incision is sutured together in a Y-shape, thus accomplishing the desired lengthening of tissue.

2.024 Rotation Flap Technique

This flap (cf. Fig. 8) is a modified form of the advancement flap technique (von Burow [212,213]). The incision line on the short side of the excised part is not extended in a linear direction, but rather in an arc shape. Here as well, one or several Burow triangles are excised on the contralateral side of the incision [cf. 140,344,352]. After the skin areas lying between the excision site and incision end are undermined, they are shifted into the primary operation defect, which is then closed free of tension.

Preferred region of application: scalp, eyelids, cheeks, lips, neck, and trunk.

2.025 Transposition Flap Technique

The principle of this method (cf. Fig.

9) is that after excision of the focus, a pedicled flap is transposed from the surrounding area into the round- to oblong-shaped operation defect. The donor site of the flap is closed by primary suture [64,127,219,354,442,443].

Preferred regions permitting favorable postoperative results: nose, eyelids, in the pre- and postauricular region, and neck and trunk area. This technique is especially recommended for postradiation injuries.

2.026 Island Flap Technique

With this method, tissue defect is closed by a subcutaneous pedicled flap from the surrounding area. The pedicle contains the vessels supplying blood (cf. Figs. 34 and 68).

Preferred region of application: nose and ear.

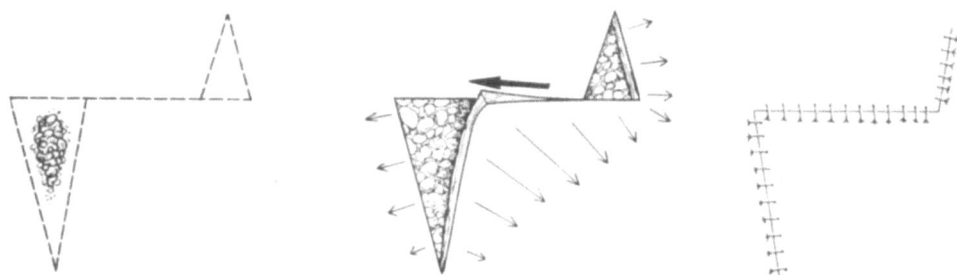

Fig. 7. *Advancement flap technique* (according to von Burow).

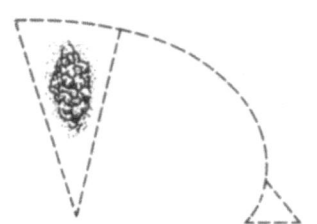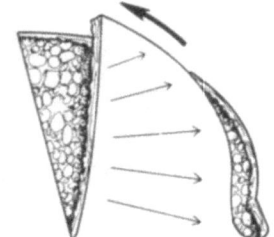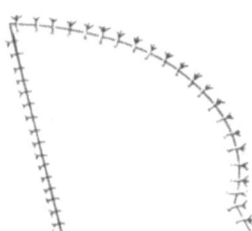

Fig. 8. *Rotation flap technique.*

2.027 Combination of Techniques

The previously mentioned techniques may be combined when dealing with relatively large defects.

Since the quality of the transplanted skin area is largely the same for local flap grafts as that at the excision site, favorable cosmetic results are likely. When dealing with hair-bearing skin components, hair lines and the direction of hair growth must be considered as much as possible.

2.028 Flaps and Grafts from Other Body Areas

2.029 Free Skin Grafts

Essential prerequisites for the adherence of free skin grafts are a good hemostasis, the avoidance of coarse ligatures, a wound bed with sufficient vascular supply, and most of all, an optimal bandaging technique (Georg [156]). Light pressure should be applied to establish a direct contact between the graft and its nourishing base. If free grafts lie in the vicinity of joints (extremities or neck, for instance), immobilization by means of a split or plaster of Paris cast [92] is recommended.

1. Full-thickness skin grafts (Wolfe-Krause [cf. 6,20,245,418,420,421,504]): The full-thickness skin to be transplanted is best prepared manually according to the exact area required. The advantages of this type of free skin graft are the minimal likelihood of shrinkage and the ability of the grafts to withstand pressure. One disadvantage, however, is that if a capillary hemorrhage occurs in the wound bed, complete or partial graft necrosis is possible. If the wound bed has been appropriately prepared, full-thickness skin grafts heal relatively well in re-

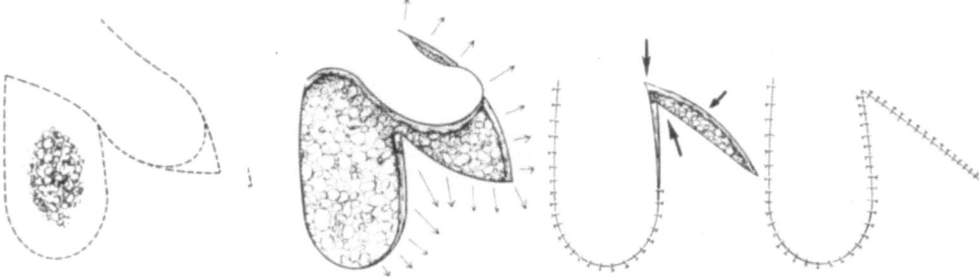

Fig. 9. *Transposition flap technique.*

gions over flat bones and on a surface which is firm and fairly smooth (craniofacially, scalp, extremities). In contrast to pedicled flaps, the scars in this case almost never enlarge since, as a rule, there is no tension [472].

2. *Split-thickness skin grafts:* The advantage of split-thickness skin, usually removed by means of a dermatome, is the substantially smaller risk of a necrosis, when compared to the fullthickness skin graft. However, its tendency to shrink, observed even after postoperative application of bandages for immobilization [498], prohibits its application in body regions which are exposed to greater stress. The aesthetic result on visible sites is not optimal, but the technique is ideal for repairing varicose ulcers and large defects which are corrected by prostheses [29,46,80].

3. *Punch grafts (Reverdin[392]):* this method involves the grafting of small cutis or split-thickness skin patches of up to roughly 1 cm (½ in.) in diameter. Their application in dermatosurgery is limited to defect repair of small ulcers, because of their poor cosmetic results.

2.030 Tubed Pedicled Flaps

In this procedure, a pedicled flap consisting of epidermis, cutis, and subcutis is brought into a surgical defect from another site, either directly (cf., among others [234,291,315,395]) or in several steps (jump graft). If possible, the remainder of the pedicled flap should be returned to the donor site during another session. Plastic surgery, which requires tubed pedicled flaps, is technically difficult, requires a great deal of time, and generally exceeds the competence of dermatosurgery. Optimal curative and aesthetic results are achieved in dermatosurgery with the

methods of local flaps and autologous skin grafts. Because the skin transplanted by local flaps is very similar in structure and function to that which is excised [cf. 194,254], local flaps are preferred to free skin grafts whenever possible. It is important, however, to observe the hair conditions in the donor and receiver areas [206]. Free grafts are recommended, especially if there is insufficient material available for local graft, for example, on the extremities and possibly the nose.

2.031 Dermabrasion

This treatment was introduced to dermatosurgery by Kromeyer [249] [cf. also 104,362,364,471] and signified great therapeutic progress when compared to techniques practiced earlier, such as cauterization, decortication (Dubreuilh), or even radiation [cf. 485].

Dermabrasion requires the use of electrically powered rotary instruments, the number of revolutions of which has been increased to 30,000–35,000 rpm at the suggestion of Schreus [437]. This increase in rpm greatly facilitates the abrasion of tissue when compared to old equipment with a speed of only 3000–6000 rpm. The number of revolutions on the modern appliances is automatically adjustable by means of a foot switch. Ruby, diamond, and metal fraises and rotating nylon and wire brushes are used for planing. In order to prevent disturbing scars, dermabrasion beyond the epidermis-cutis border must be avoided, unless scarring is considered of secondary importance, for example, in the removal of tattoos [414]. When foreign body intrusions [cf. also 307] lie partially in the bottom layers of the corium or subcutis, good cosmetic results are achieved [470] by combining high-speed dermabrasion (to eradicate superficial lesions) and punching for the deep deposits, where the punch wounds are primarily sutured.

The danger of pigment displacement due to sun exposure after high-speed dermabrasion is avoided, for the most part, by scheduling the operations for fall and winter months [438].

2.032 Electrosurgery

A high-frequency surgical appliance must be available for this method. The basic principal in electrosurgery is that a high-frequency current is conducted from a large-area neutral electrode over the patient's body to a small-area active electrode. In the process, a high current density is reached in the active electrode which, as minimum values are exceeded, causes the required heating necessary in the tissue for coagulation or cutting. High frequency currents of 500 kHz are necessary to prevent faradic irritation of nerves and musculature.

2.033 Electrotomy

This process refers to the electrocaustic penetration of tissue. For smooth incisions without superficial coagulation, needle or lancet electrodes of the thinnest possible cross section are most suitable. Since wounds caused by electric current tend to heal slowly, it is advisable in tumor surgery to perform skin incisions with the scalpel and then continue the operation with the electric knife. When removing verrucae vulgaris electrocaustically, it is likewise advisable to first peritomize it by means of a scalpel with a 2–3 mm (¼ in.) margin and then excise it with the electric loop (for technique cf. [102,106]). During this procedure the extirpation must not be made too deep into the corium, or else unattractive scars will result [474].

2.034 Coagulation

All types of active electrodes can be used for this process of cauterizing tissue—for example, fine needle electrodes for epilation, and ball and plate electrodes for closure of hemorrhaging vessels and capillaries. It is important that the surface of the electrodes is always kept clean since a crust composed of burned tissue and blood remnants isolates the electrode surface and can lead to sparking and charring of the contact area.

2.035 Desiccation

Desiccation means the drying-up of tissue in the immediate area around an inserted electrode due to coagulation. This method cannot be monitored by the naked eye; therefore inexperienced use could result in extensive tissue necrosis [cf. e.g., 167,487].

2.036 Fulguration

In this method an arc from a high-voltage electrode causes the burning of the skin surface. Since carbonization and necrosis are common results of this procedure, it is no longer used very frequently.

2.037 Curettage

This procedure involves the excision of cutaneous lesions (for example, verrucae seborrhoicae) with the aid of a curette. An active hemostasis is not generally necessary.

2.038 Chemosurgery

The technique in use today was listed by Mohs [302,303] as an improvement of Schreus' zinc-chloride cautery for epitheliomas. After curettage or excision of the tumor, zinc-chloride fixative is applied to the tumor bed and the tissue, and when affixed is excised parallel to the surface. This procedure must be repeated several times until tumor tissue is not detected histologically.

Having only little personal experience with this method of treatment, we refer to the numerous publications dealing with it (survey in [47], cf. also [273,301,366,482].

3. Special Techniques for Different Regions of the Body

3.001 Scalp

A good cosmetic result is frequently achieved by an advancement or rotation flap when primary wound suturing is impossible on the scalp. A free transplant must be considered only when the excisions are large in area and the general condition of the patient is poor. As a rule, the excision of malignant and semimalignant neoplasms extends to the periosteum, but if proven necessary (in dermatofibrosarcoma protuberans, for instance,) it too can be removed without risk [56]. To assure optimal vascular supply, the skin areas to be transplanted are cut together with the galea down to the periosteum and transposed. Interrupted sutures (suture material of the strength 0–0 to 1–0) are used for wound closure; atraumatic suture material is not required. Because of the danger of profuse bleeding during extensive operations in the scalp area, prior determination of blood type and a preoperative physical examination are indispensable (coagulation disorder due to loss of blood).

3.002 Rotation Flap Technique

After triangular excision of the focus, the incision along the triangle's short side is continued dorsolaterally or dorsomedially to form an arc. One or several Burow triangles on the contralateral side of the incision are excised. After undermining, the skin area lying between the excision site and the Burow triangle is transposed into the operation defect and sutured without tension [cf. Fig. 10].

3.003 Double Rotation Flap Technique

In contrast to simple rotation flaps, two arc-shaped incisions are continued in opposite directions from two diametrically opposed points on the defect. One or several Burow triangles must be excised on the contralateral side of the incisions. The skin areas defined by both incisions are undermined and then shifted in opposite directions so that a reasonably tension-free wound closure results (cf. Fig. 11, Plate 1).

3.004 Rotation Flap Technique Combined with Free Skin Graft

This method is recommended for larger surgical defects that cannot be closed by a double rotation flap technique, particularly those resulting from removal of radiation ulcers [512].

The preparation of the flap to be

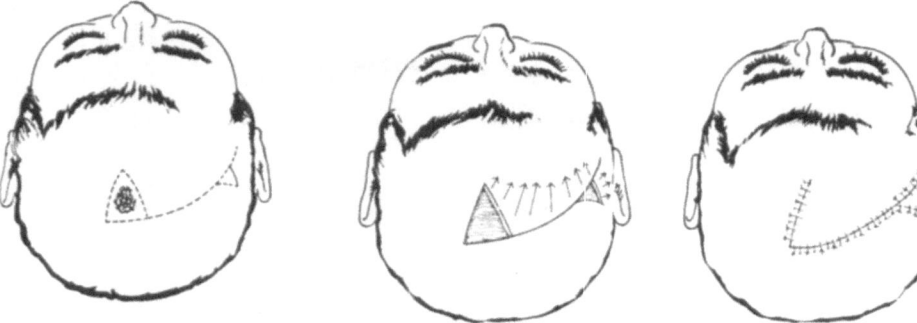

Fig. 10. *Rotation flap technique.*

transplanted follows the same procedure as for the simple rotation flap technique. The secondary defect is repaired
with a free full-thickness skin graft after
exact hemostasis ([193], cf. also Fig.
12). If the graft is extensive, it is perforated to facilitate drainage of secretion and is best taken from the thigh
with an electrodermatome.

3.005 Full-Thickness Skin Graft

If extensive surgery seems unadvis-
able due to the general condition of the
patient, the defect can be repaired by
a full-thickness skin graft [156]. This
method is advisable even when there is
no hair on the scalp and when a cosmetically superior result cannot be
achieved by a rotation flap.

3.006 Transplantation of Multiple Punch Biopsies

The method of transplanting multiple
punch biopsies from hair-bearing skin
[99,334] is suitable for treating circumscribed baldness, particularly in the
temple area. Its application to correct
androgenic alopecia, however, does
not always yield satisfactory cosmetic
results [137,484,488].

3.007 Surgery for Relaxation of the Scalp

Final results are likewise unsatisfactory in this operation ("epicraniotomy"
[135,493]). The galea aponeurotica of
the forehead is separated in its entire
width above a 15–20 mm incision in the

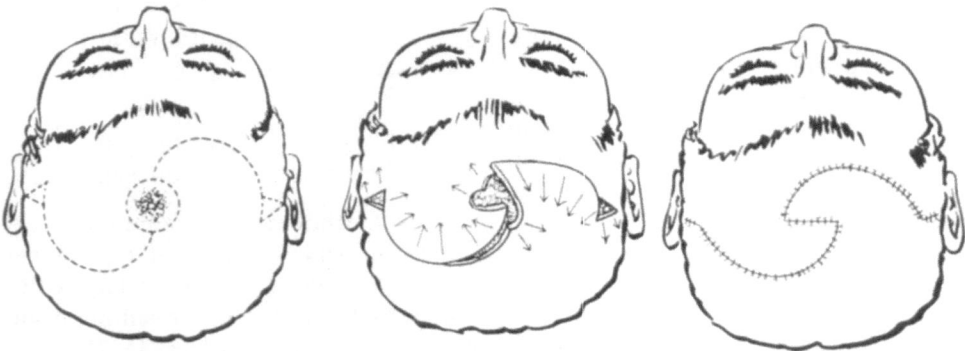

Fig. 11. *Double rotation flap technique.*

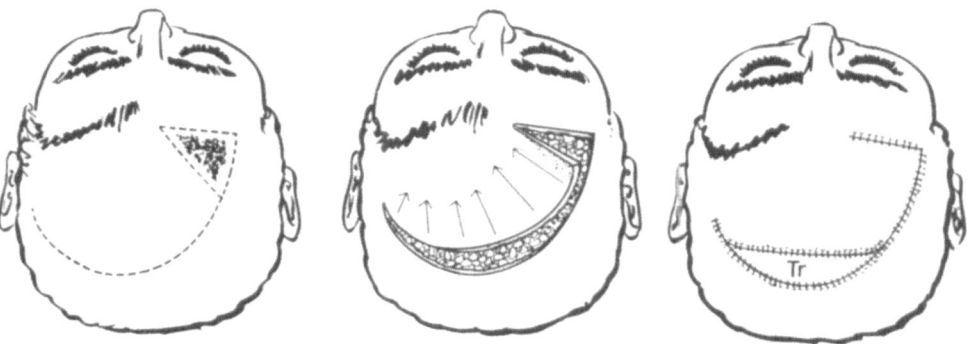

Fig. 12. *Rotation flap technique combined with freeskin graft.* TR: skin graft.

eyebrows or a thumb's width above them (Bruck [43]) and the galea is at least partially removed. In some of his patients, Bruck saw a marked improvement of the condition; however, even he points out that the presurgical condition reappears at the latest 5 years after the operation. In addition, the success of the operation is greatly minimized by hematomas which may appear postoperatively.

3.008 Temporal Region

Here too, the methods of local flap grafting provide optimal surgical results [344,345], and because of the favorable vascular supply, the danger of partial flap necrosis is relatively slight even for the grafting of larger skin segments.

3.009 Caudal Advancement Flap Technique

A triangular excision of the focus is made so that the short side of the triangle is placed supraauricularly. The short side of the triangle is then extended preauricularly to the maxillofacial corner. This incision lies in a preformed crease. A Burow triangle is then excised below the ear. After the skin lying between the excision site and the Burow triangle is undermined, it is shifted upward to cover the defect (Fig. 13, Plate 2). When mobilizing subcutaneously as well as when making an in-

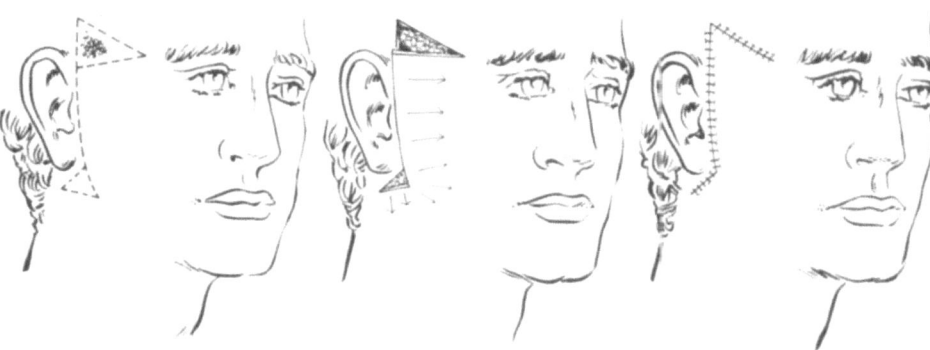

Fig. 13. *Caudal advancement flap technique.*

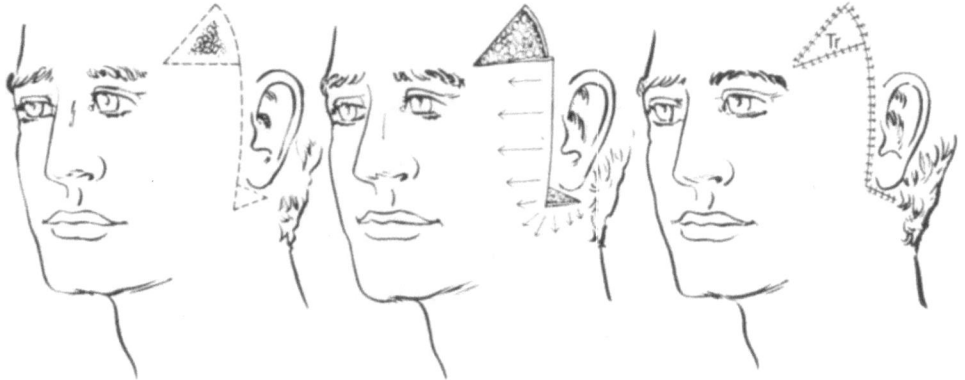

Fig. 14. *Advancement flap technique—combined with free skin graft.* TR: skin graft.

cision preauricularly, the directions of the facial nerves must be observed (Fig. 2) so as to avoid peripheral facial paralysis.

3.010 Advancement Flap Technique–Free Skin Grafting Combination

If a surgical defect cannot be closed by the advancement or rotation flap techniques alone, repair of the remaining defect is possible with a free, autologous, full-thickness skin graft from the inner side of the upper arm (Fig. 14).

3.011 Dorsal Rotation Flap Technique

This technique is used to repair surgical defects in the hair-bearing region of the temples. The skin is advanced along an arc-shaped incision, extending from the defect to the back of the head. A Burow triangle is then excised contralaterally to the incision line (cf. Fig. 15).

3.012 Caudal Rotation Flap Technique

This technique may also be considered for repairing a defect in the hair-

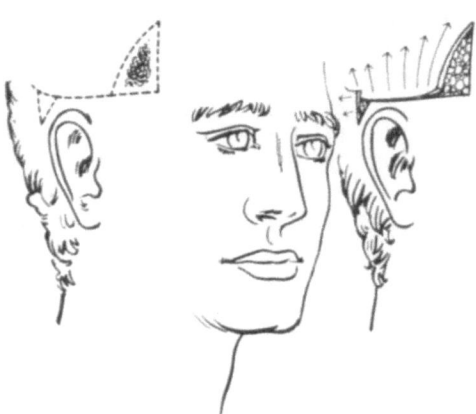
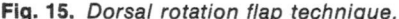
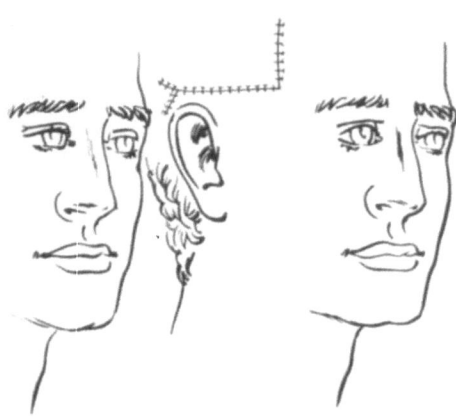

Fig. 15. *Dorsal rotation flap technique.*

bearing temple region (cf. Fig. 16). As for all other regional flaps in the scalp and temple region, continuous suction by means of plastic tubing should always be used.

3.013 Free Skin Grafting Technique (Split-thickness Skin Grafts)

This technique may be preferred if malignant tumors were not excised in toto and/or the defect must be monitored for recurrence.

3.014 Forehead

The osseous skull itself sets limits to primary wound closure even after undermining of the wound edges in medium-sized defects. The forehead is the region of the head best suited to free grafts, for the deviating structure of the donor site is least noticeable here. If, however, free autologous skin is not used for repair, a local flap will also provide satisfying results.

3.015 Rotation Flap Technique

After the focus is localized in the lateral third of the forehead, a triangle-shaped excision is made, followed by an arc-shaped incision conforming to the hair line and proceeding over the preformed preauricular creases up to the maxillofacial corner. A Burow triangle is made below the ear on the contralateral side of the incision. The skin segments lying between the excision site and the Burow triangle are carefully prepared and rotated into the surgical defect (cf. Fig. 17). If the defect cannot be closed completely by this method, the remainder is repaired as in the temporal region with free autologous skin or by a frontal rotation flap (cf. also Plate 3).

3.016 Advancement Flap Technique from Both Temporal Areas

If the focus lies in the middle of the forehead, the surgical defect is repaired by an advancement of the lateral skin segments of the forehead. In this procedure, the first incision is made in the

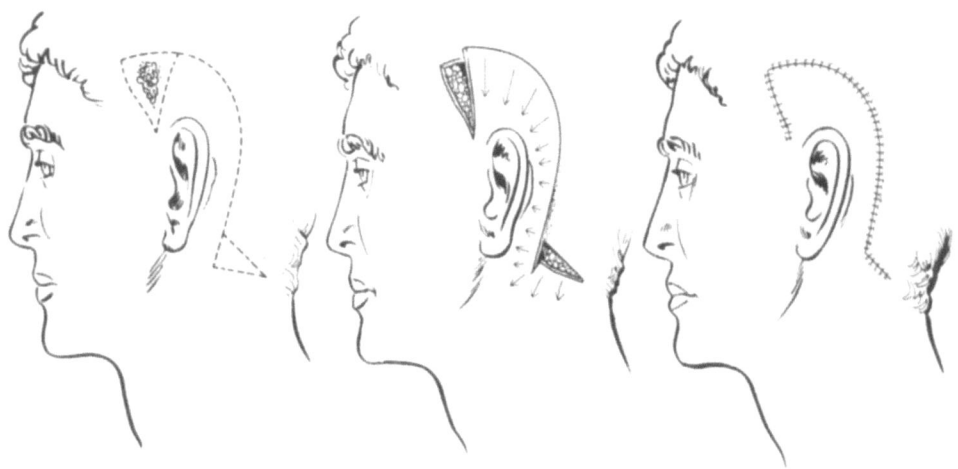

Fig. 16. *Caudal rotation flap technique.*

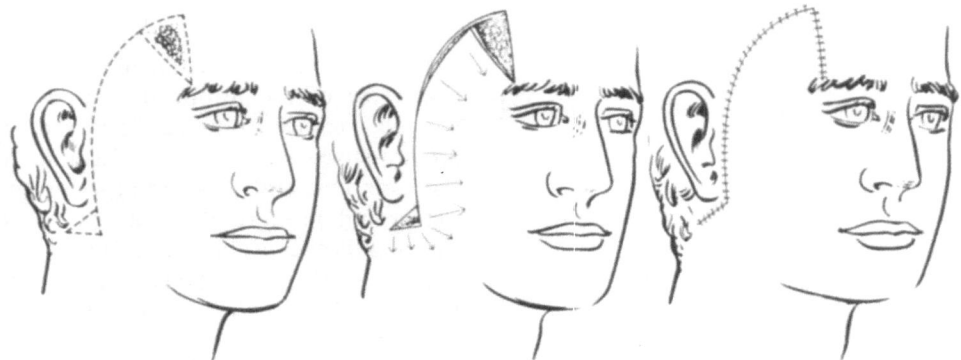

Fig. 17. *Rotation flap technique* in the lateral forehead.

region of the hairline on the forehead, the other, above the eyebrows. Burow triangles are made in the temporal area at both ends of the two incisions. After the skin segments lying between the excision site and Burow triangles are mobilized, they are advanced medially, thus closing the defect (Fig. 18, also called U-flap technique.)

3.017 Double Rotation Flap

When there are large tissue losses in the midforehead, this method can effect a largely tension-free wound closure. Starting from the ends of the oval defect, two arc-shaped incisions are made in opposite directions. One incision proceeds along the hairline and the

other along the eyebrow, both in the direction of the temporal regions, where Burow triangles are excised contralaterally to the excision sites. The peritomized forehead skin is then mobilized and shifted medially (Fig. 19, Plate 4).

3.018 Nose

Careful planning is especially important when operating in the nasal region [42,73,75,95,219,234,238,457]. Even a slight nasal deviation can cause functional disorders, such as a blocking of the nasal passage [320]. An aesthetically dissatisfying postoperative result

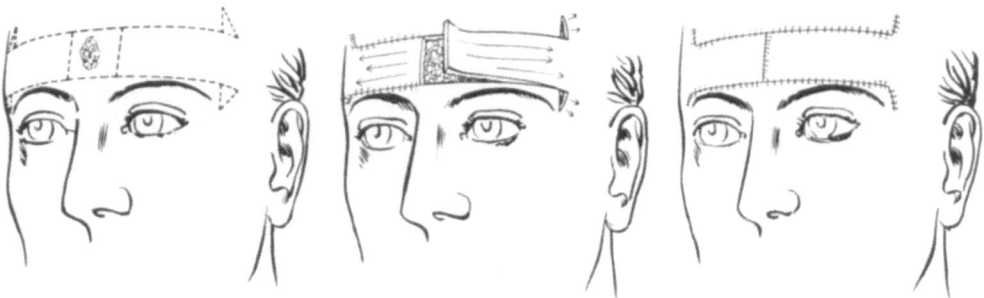

Fig. 18. *Advancement flap technique from both temporal areas.*

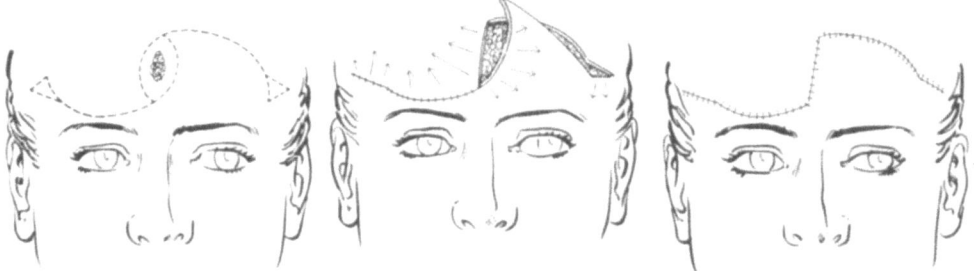

Fig. 19. *Double rotation flap technique* for defects in the medial forehead.

as a rule means disfigurement of the patient [319,358,373].

When a tumor is present, the treatment must completely eradicate the neogenesis, yet spare the surrounding healthy tissue as much as possible [281]. Therefore, particularly on the nose, surgery is superior to radiation [347]; due to anatomic structures here, the danger of causing radiation injuries to the skin and to the cartilage lying directly beneath it is especially great.

Frequently, in order to achieve a primary wound closure, too small a safety margin is maintained due to the special nasal topography; this results in a large number of tumor recurrences. Excision is successful only if made far enough into the healthy tissue, but a primary suture is possible for only very small defects. If a disfiguring distortion of the nose is to be avoided, plastic repair of the defect proves necessary especially for children and for injuries resulting from X-rays [73,74].

3.019 Transposition Flap Technique

A focus located in the ala nasi may be excised far into the healthy tissue and the resulting defect repaired by means of a transposition flap from the nasolabial region. The flap donor site is sutured primarily so that the resultant surgical scar rests in the nasolabial crease and will be unnoticeable later (cf. Fig. 20, Plate 5).

This technique can be used if the mucous membrane remains intact or if only small surgical defects result which are treated with primary catgut suture. Larger defects in the mucous membrane are closed by skin flaps from the surrounding area in the form of transposition or island flaps [73].

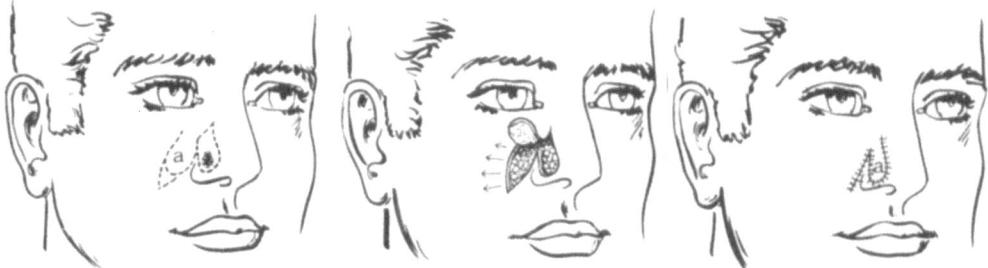

Fig. 20. *Transposition flap technique* for defects of the ala nasi (mucous membrane intact).

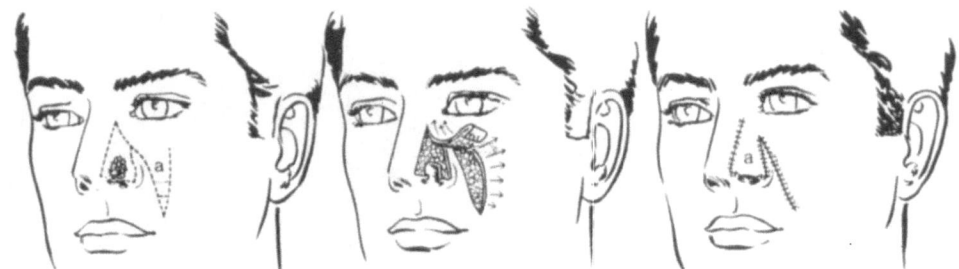

Fig. 21. *Transposition flap technique* on the ala nasi for a large penetrating defect.

When there are extensive defects on the ala nasi with loss of mucous membrane and cartilage components, a sufficiently large transposition flap can be shifted from the nasolabial region into the operation defect [486] by turning the distal flap component inward to form the inner lining of the nose (Fig. 21, Plate 6).

Smaller excision wounds on the nasal tip can also be repaired occasionally by a simple transposition flap from the ala nasi [276] which is then closed by Dehnungsplastik. When defects are present on the dorsum nasi, the double transposition flap may also be used [312], the second flap being removed from the forehead (cf. Fig. 23).

3.020 Double Transposition Flap Technique

A surgical defect in the area of the nasal tip may be closed by a double transposition flap procedure [cf. 91]. First, the wound on the nasal tip is closed by means of a transposition flap from the ala nasi; its donor site is closed with a transposition flap from the nasolabial crease. This donor site is sutured primarily and is unnoticeable due to its location (Fig. 22, Plate 7).

3.021 Lateral Advancement Flap Technique

The focus is excised in the shape of a triangle within the healthy tissue. The incision in the area of the short side of the triangle is extended in a lateral direction and a Burow triangle made on the contralateral side in the nasolabial crease. After the skin segment lying between the excision site and the Burow triangle is undermined, it is shifted into the surgical defect and closed free

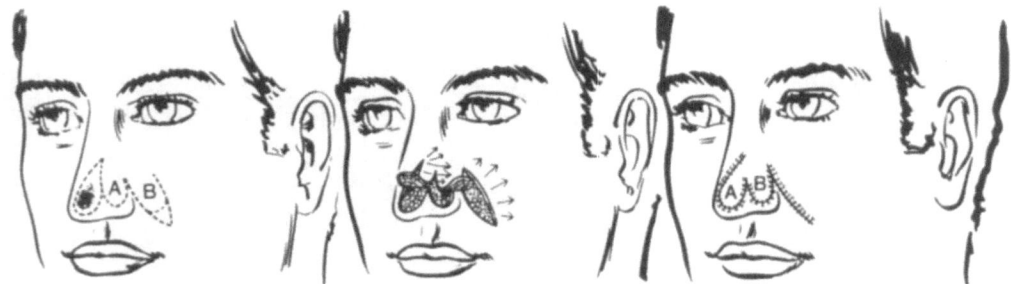

Fig. 22. *Double transposition flap technique* for a defect on the tip of the nose.

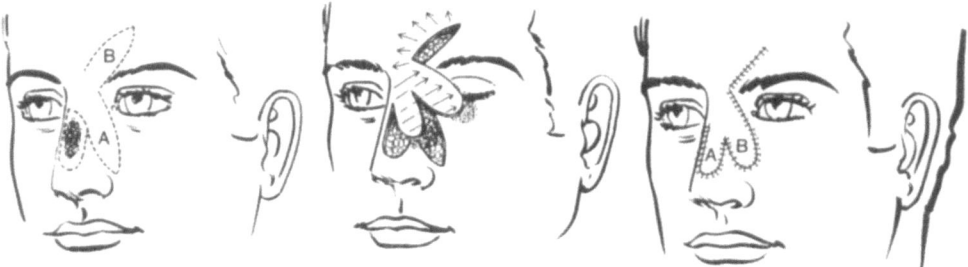

Fig. 23. *Double transposition flap technique* for defects on the dorsum nasi.

of tension. This technique allows the additional scar resulting from the operation to also rest in the nasolabial crease (Fig. 24). If defects are larger, it is possible to close them by shifting the skin laterally from both sides (double advancement flap, Fig. 25).

3.022 Cranial Advancement Flap Technique

The focus is extirpated in the form of a square, the two perpendicular sides of which are extended by vertical incisions as far as the glabella, where a Burow triangle is made laterally on each incision. The peritomized strip of tissue is placed in the defect after mobilizing the forehead skin (Fig. 26, also called U-flap technique).

3.023 Caudal Advancement Flap Technique

After triangular removal of the focus in the ala nasi, the short side of the triangle is continued caudally in the shape of an "S" and a half-moon-shaped skin segment is excised from the nasolabial crease. After undermining the skin area to be transposed, it is shifted into the primary defect in the direction of the cranium, thus allowing a tension-free wound closure (Fig. 27). The procedure is the same for defects of the inner canthus.

3.024 Rotation Flap Technique for Defects of Ala Nasi

This procedure is an alternative to the caudal advancement flap technique. After vertical, triangular excision of a

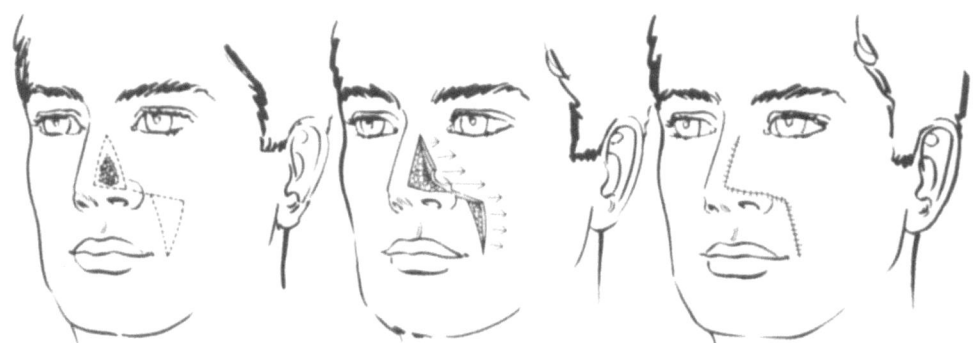

Fig. 24. *Lateral advancement flap technique* for a defect of the ala nasi.

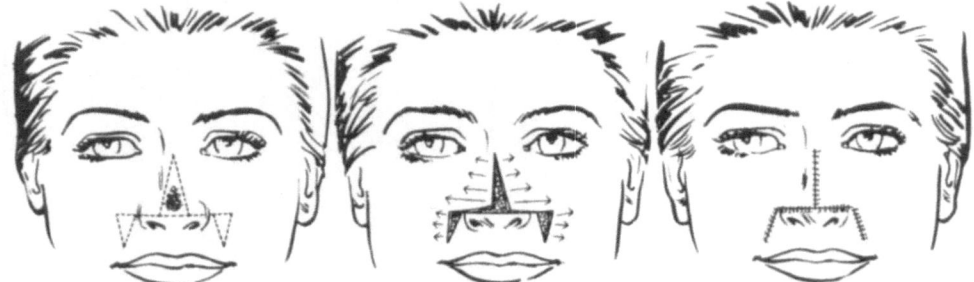

Fig. 25. *Double lateral advancement flap technique* for a defect of the dorsum nasi and tip.

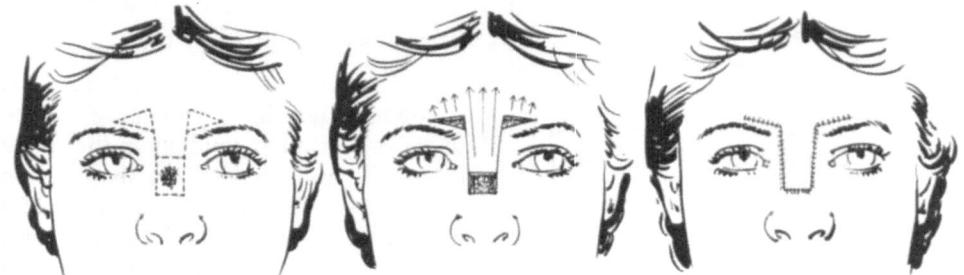

Fig. 26. *Cranial advancement flap technique* for a defect of the dorsum nasi.

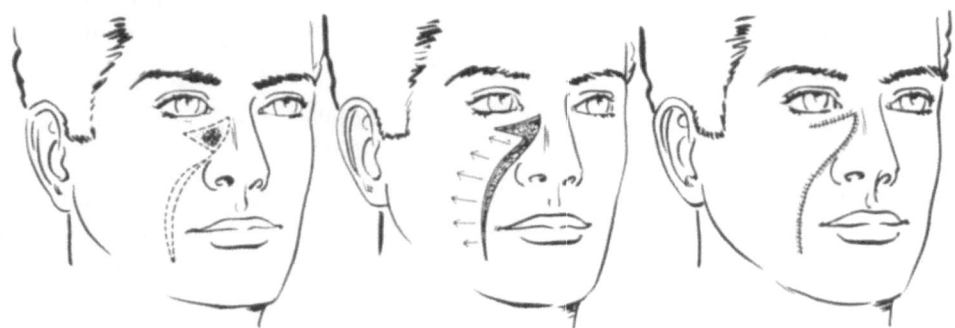

Fig. 27. *Caudal advancement flap technique* in the lateral nose area.

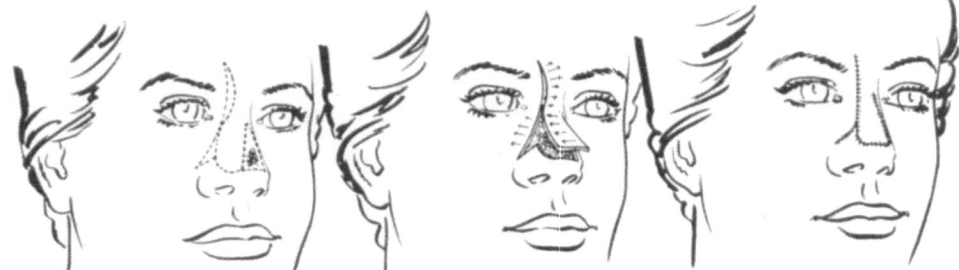

Fig. 28. *Rotation flap technique* for defects of ala nasi.

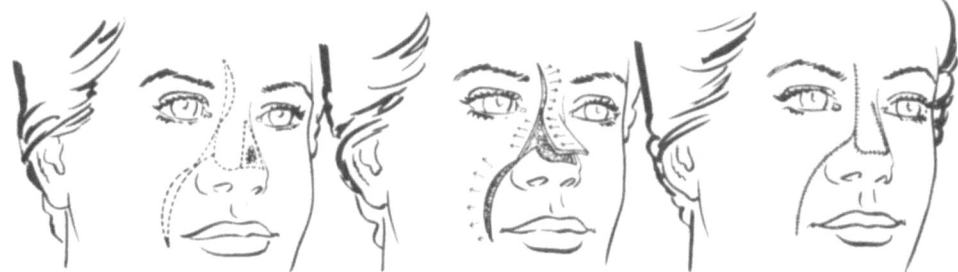

Fig. 29. *Rotation flap technique* combined with caudal advancement flap for defects of ala nasi.

focus, the short side of the triangle is extended by an arc-shaped incision over the contralateral side of the nose to the glabella, where a crescent-shaped skin segment is excised. A Burow triangle is also excised contralaterally in the nasolabial crease. The peritomized skin segments can then be mobilized and rotated into the defect (Fig. 28). If a tension-free wound closure proves impossible using this procedure, a caudal advancement flap must be added (Fig. 29, Plate 8).

3.025 Rotation Flap Technique for Defects of the Nasal Tip

This procedure is combined with a VY flap in the area of the glabella [218,398]. The focus is removed horizontally in the shape of a triangle, the short side of which is extended by an arc-shaped incision to the glabella and bent there to form a "V." The peritomized skin segment is then mobilized from the base and shifted into the defect. The resulting gap in the area of the glabella is closed by a VY flap (Fig. 30, Plate 9).

3.026 Tunnel Flap Technique

When handling defects in the region of the nasal floor and the nose septum, a tunnel flap from the nasolabial region applied cranially (Fig. 31, Plate 10) or caudally (Fig. 32) yields satisfactory results. Due to its favorable vascular supply [299], this flap may be cut extremely long when there is a small base; according to Cameron et al., [50], the relationship of the base to the length may be 1:4. We are essentially dealing with a modified transposition flap (see

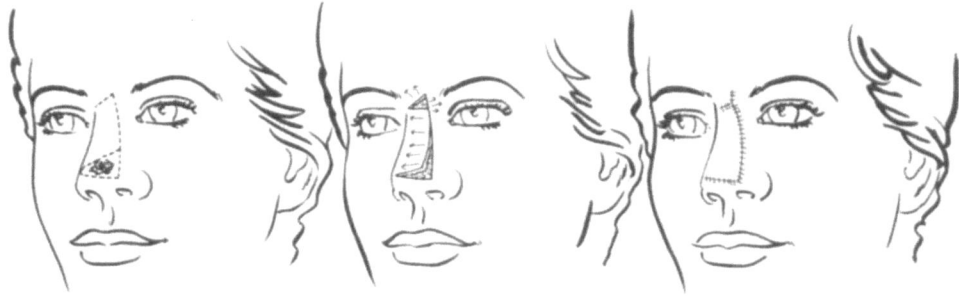

Fig. 30. *Rotation flap technique for defects of the nasal tip* combined with VY-flap in the area of the glabella.

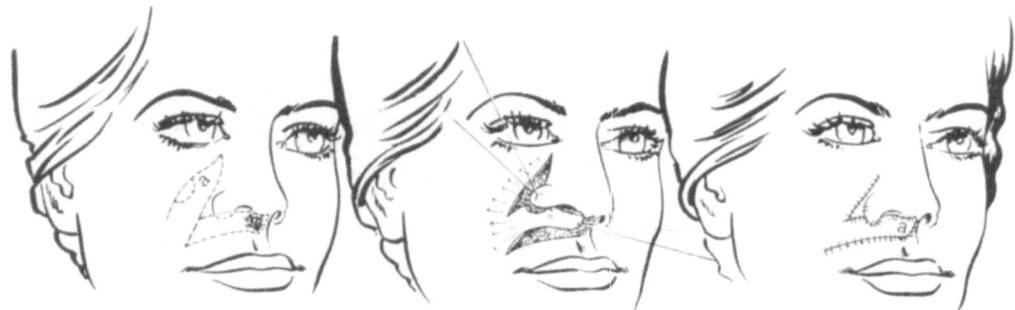

Fig. 31. *Tunnel flap technique.* Skin from the cranium is used for repairing a defect of the nasal base.

Sect. 3.019). After tunneling under ala nasi, the skin component to be transplanted is moved through this passage and into the primary operation defect [157].

3.027 Columella Nasi Reconstruction Technique

The reconstruction of the skin component of the columella is made with one or two horizontal transposition flaps from the upper lip [73]. This method is not too difficult technically and gives results that are cosmetically and functionally favorable (Fig. 33, Plate 11).

3.028 Island Flap Technique

A flap pedicled only by its vascular supply (Dunham [34], and Monks [308]) and taken from the nasolabial or cranial region may be used to repair nonpenetrating skin defects and to correct defects of the mucous membrane [109,112]. It is brought into the defect by means of a subcutaneous tunnel, and the flap donor site is sutured primarily (Fig. 34) [8].

3.029 Composite Grafts

So-called composite grafts [263,419] are suited for defects which penetrate the ala nasi or as a columella replacement. Using the auricle as the donor site (Fig. 35), the secondary defect of the auricle is closed either primarily, as is done after making a triangular excision, or in the manner of a Trendelenburg flap (see Sect. 3.060). Likewise a shortening of the ala nasi, often resulting from an accident, is corrected with the aid of a composite graft [486].

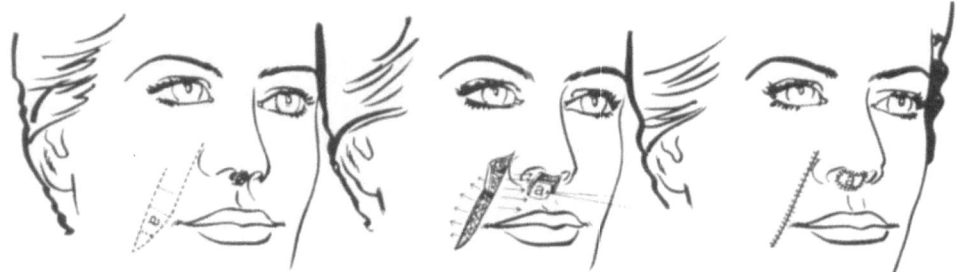

Fig. 32. *Caudal tunnel flap technique* for the closure of a defect of the nasal base.

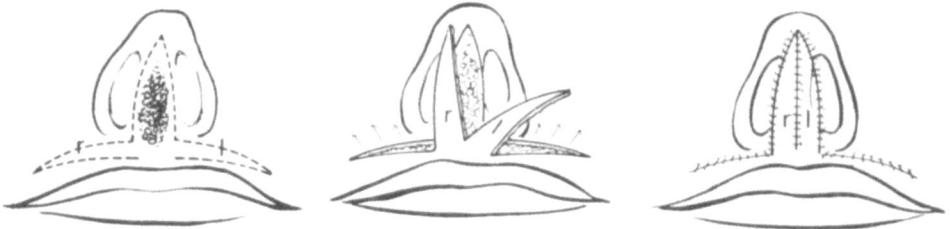

Fig. 33. *Columella reconstruction technique* using double transposition flap (flap donor site: upper lip).

3.030 Z-Flap Technique

This method frequently achieves better cosmetic results than the implantation of composite grafts (Fig. 36) in the case of less-pronounced deformities of the ala nasi.

3.031 Free Skin Grafting

Obviously free skin grafts can also be used in the nasal area (cf. also Petres 1969 [347,349]), but the cosmetic result depends on complete healing of the graft. Pigment displacement in the graft [63,275] may be compensated for by dermabrasion [462]. Prophylaxis consists in strictly avoiding strong sunlight for several months, possibly in conjunction with the use of sun-blocking ointments.

3.032 Rhinophyma Therapy

Rhinophyma is always treated surgically [cf. 232], excellent results being achieved by excising hyperplasia of the sebaceous glands [94,96,115,118, 130,132,219,260] with the scalpel ("decortication") and then by remodelling the nose by high-speed dermabrasion [136,249] to restore its original shape. Bleeding may be profuse, but can be ignored generally. The reepithelization of the wound areas is achieved relatively quickly from the epithelium of the sebaceous glands located in the deep tissue (Plate 12).

Warning: Avoid too deep an excision which would result in a slow healing process and disturbing scar formation.

Radical excision of rhinophyma [cf. 75] and subsequent repair of the surgi-

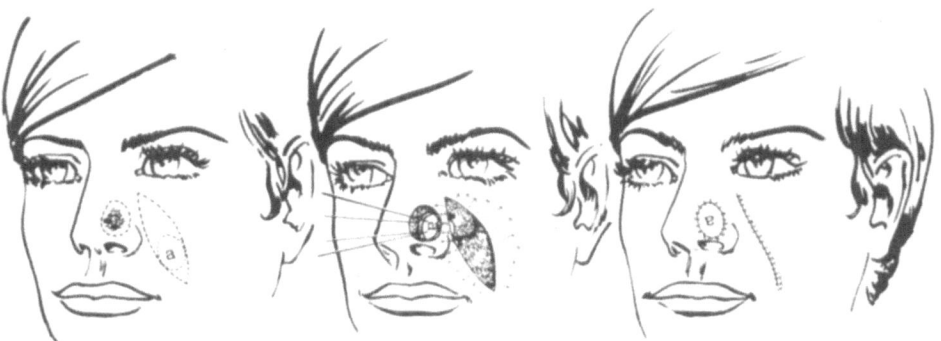

Fig. 34. *Island flap technique* for defect of the ala nasi (flap donor site: nasolabial region).

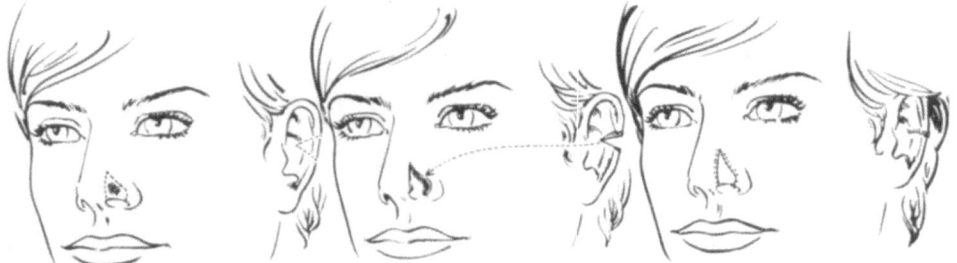

Fig. 35. *Composite graft* for penetrating defect of the ala nasi (donor site: auricle).

cal defect by free autologous skin grafts is not recommended because of unsatisfactory cosmetic results [150]. Subcutaneous extirpation [122] is not necessary since it is more complicated and the end result is aesthetically inferior to decortication.

3.033 Lips

Numerous surgical methods for this area have been described (cf. among others [61,62,155,181,183,196,199,239, 251,337,491]). Some of these methods are too extensive; others result in deformity [235,270].

If there is a precancerosis or stage I carcinoma (Eller and Eller [450]), radical excision suffices [363]. Neither a

follow-up radiation treatment nor an en bloc dissection with lymphadenectomy is necessary [129], but frequent checkups are essential [278,377]. However, the chances of a successful operation decrease if after an insufficient initial operation and previous radiation treatment a recurring tumor is suspected [233].

Only those methods will be described below which are technically uncomplicated and from which favorable results, both curative and aesthetic, can be expected.

3.034 Vermilionectomy for the Lower Lip (Langenbeck and von Bruns)

This method [44,259] is recommended for precancerous neoplasm and carcinomas of the lower lip which have

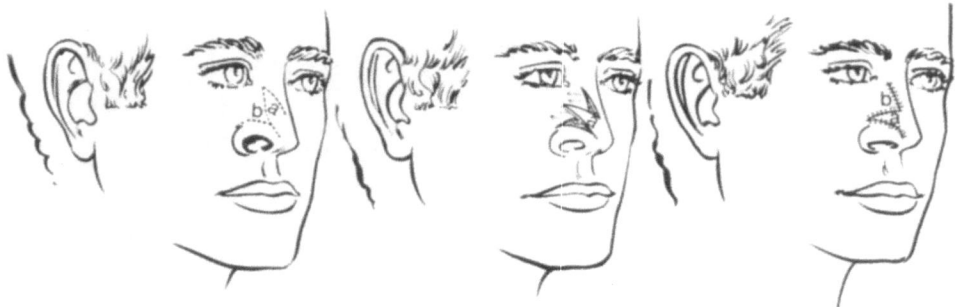

Fig. 36. *Z-flap technique* for shortening of the ala nasi.

not yet progressed beyond the border of the labium [45,48,184,253,269,351, 463]; it does not necessarily require hospitalization. The operation is performed under local anesthesia [144], the injection of which proceeds from the corners of the mouth, so that the lip protrudes. An anesthetic mixed with epinephrine is recommended since this mixture minimizes the bleeding from the extremely vascularized tissue. The patient must be made aware beforehand that the profuse bleeding is of no consequence.

A swab is placed between the teeth and the lip and the head is raised. Using only a scalpel and a small surgical forceps, the focus is excised to the necessary depth together with the entire labium. The mucous membrane of the lower lip is mobilized afterwards with dissecting scissors or a scalpel. Skin and mucous membrane edges are connected by atraumatic sutures, and the suture lines form the new border for the labium. In making the first incisions, the original shape of the labium must be considered. After abatement of any postoperative edemas which may occur, the labium is not, as a rule, substantially narrower than before. Half of the sutures are removed after 3 days; the rest, after 1 week. Special advantages of this procedure (Fig. 37) are its simplicity, minimal technical requirements, little discomfort to the patient,

and normally unproblematic healing with functional and cosmetically attractive results (Plates 13,14).

Since carcinomas of the lower lip almost never appear on unchanged labial mucosa [323] but, on occasion, even appear at several sites simultaneously [511], excision of the entire lower labium considerably decreases the danger of the carcinoma's recurrence or of a recurrence in the vicinity of the primary tumor [351].

3.035 Triangular Excision

Triangular excision (Dieffenbach [75,76] may be considered (cf. Fig. 38) for neoplasms which progress beyond prolabium. If the base of the triangle does not exceed 2 cm (¾ in.) [252], the focus is excised triangularly under local anesthesia in the healthy tissue and the wound is closed afterward layer by layer [129,133]. This method can also be applied to the upper lip. If the remaining prolabium still shows preblastomatous lesions, a lower lip transplantation according to Langenbeck and von Bruns is used during the same session [16].

Triangular excision is not suitable for tumors that are very wide since it can lead to asymmetry and constriction of the mouth. In such cases more extensive surgical techniques must be used.

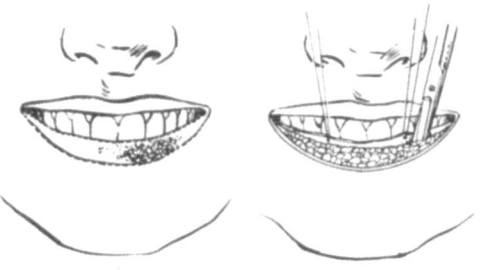
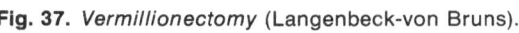
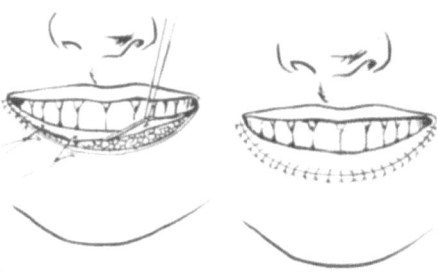

Fig. 37. *Vermillionectomy* (Langenbeck-von Bruns).

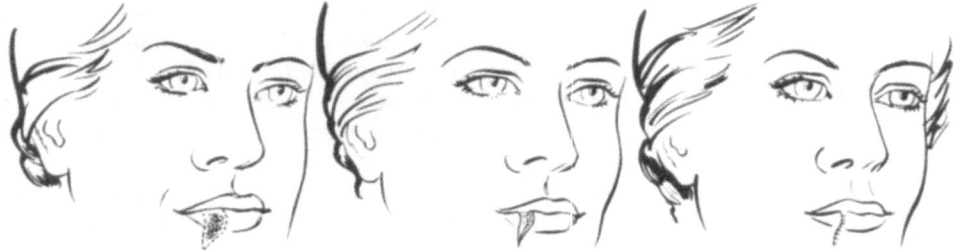

Fig. 38. *Triangular excision* of the lower lip.

3.036 Advancement Flap Techniques for the Lower Lip (von Burow)

This method can be used for extensive tumors [21]. The focus is excised according to the method described by Dieffenbach for triangular excision. Then an arc-shaped incision is made from one or both corners of the mouth toward the ear lobe, and an equilateral triangle excised from the cheek over this incision line. After undermining and uniting the wound edges in the cheek area, the sutures are placed in the nasolabial crease and the underside is simultaneously shifted medially, allowing reconstruction of the lower lip.

In the case of extensive mucous membrane defects, it may also be necessary to move cheek and buccal mucous membrane medially. In order to accomplish this the mucous membrane including the underlying soft parts is separated from the lower mandible and extended by vertical incision until a tension-free wound closure in the chin is possible [148,353]. The new lower labium is reconstructed after mobilizing the oral mucous membrane (Langenbeck and von Bruns). A wound closure is made layer by layer in the area around the triangular excision (Fig. 39).

3.037 Lower Lip Repair (Estlander)

This technique can be used on the upper as well as the lower lip [113]. The focus is excised in the shape of a triangle and the defect repaired with a transposition flap from the opposite lip. Wound closure is made layer by layer at the donor and graft sites (Fig. 40).

For neoplasms in the medial third of

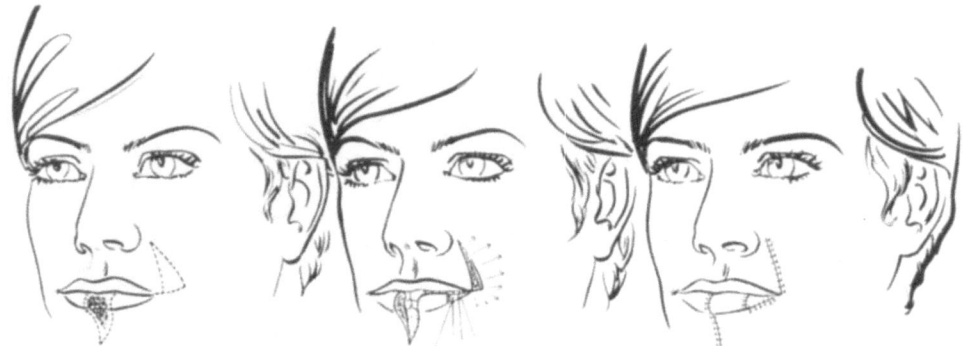

Fig. 39. *Advancement flap technique* (von Burow) for the lower lip.

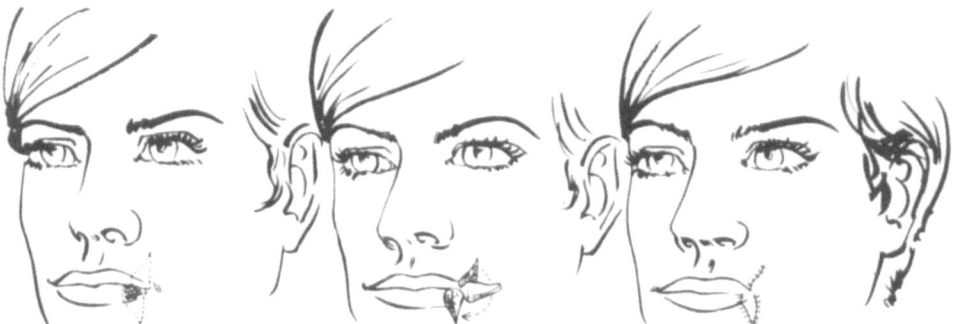

Fig. 40. *Lower lip repair (Estlander)* for defect in the lateral third of the lower lip.

the lip, a modification is necessary: the primary surgical defect is sutured layer by layer. The shortening of the lip thus caused is compensated for by making a vertical incision at the corner of the mouth and implanting the Estlander flap of the one lip into the other lip (Fig. 47). Although Estlander's technique causes a distortion of the mouth's corner, it can be corrected during a second session by means of plastic surgery to elongate the lip (see Sect. 3.040).

3.038 Transposition Flap Technique for Defects of the Lower Lip

Another possibility for repairing larger defects in the lower lip area is the use of a transposition flap from the nasolabial region [55,286]. In so doing, the buccal mucous membrane of the lips and the lower labium is reconstructed by transposing mucous membrane from the inside of the cheek (cf. Fig. 42, Plate 15).

3.039 VY-Flap Technique

A loss of substance in the medial third of the lower lip is closed by double VY-flaps without, however, shortening the lip. In this procedure, the mucous membrane of the lower lip must be mobilized along the entire width and depth of the vestibulum oris in order to direct it medially and outward. The wound is closed layer by layer.

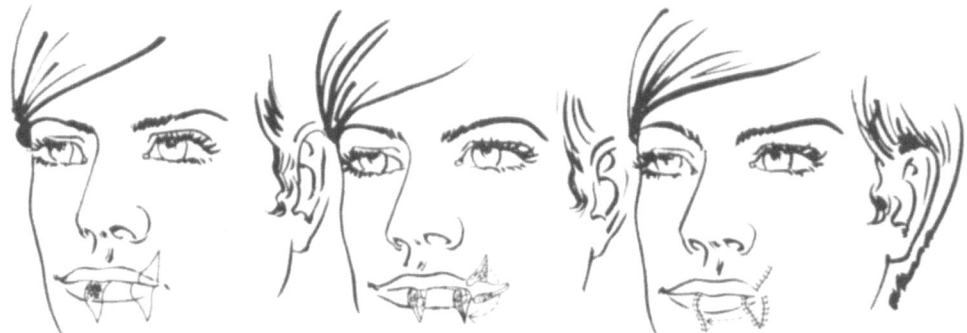

Fig. 41. *Lower lip repair (Estlander)* for the repair of a defect in the medial third of the lower lip.

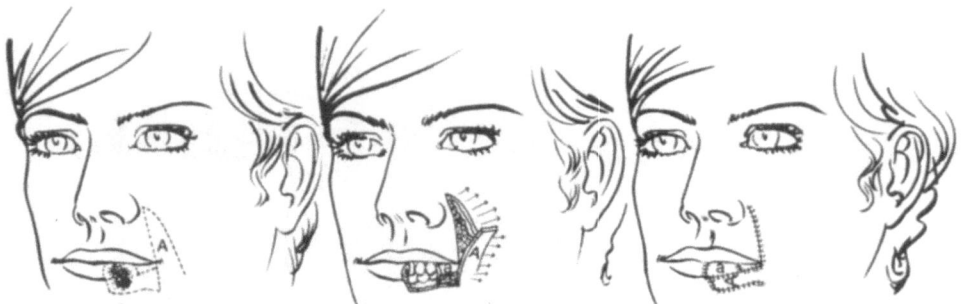

Fig. 42. *Transposition flap technique for defects of the lower lip.*

3.040 Plastic Surgery to Widen the Mouth

Performed on one side, this procedure corrects the condition created by Estlander's technique [4,360] (see Sect. 3.037); performed on both sides, it is indispensable for eliminating microcheilia and microstomy after an extended single triangular excision [65,155,160].

Preferred procedure: symmetry of the oral cavity is created by making an incision from the corner of the mouth on the constricted side, horizontally through all layers of the cheek. An adequate, large transposition flap dissected from the prolabium beforehand is used to reconstruct the missing lower labial component. The missing upper prolabium is formed by advancing mo- bilized mucous membrane from the upper lip or cheek (Fig. 43).

3.041 Transposition Flap Technique for Upper Lip Repair

As are cases involving the lower lip, defects of the upper lip are, if the mucous membrane remains intact, repaired with the aid of a nasolabial flap. The flap donor site is sutured primarily. If required, the prolabial component is replaced by the advancement of lip mucous membrane (Fig. 44).

3.042 Advancement Flap Technique (von Burow) for Upper Lip Repair

Large penetrating defects of the upper lip are satisfactorily treated from a

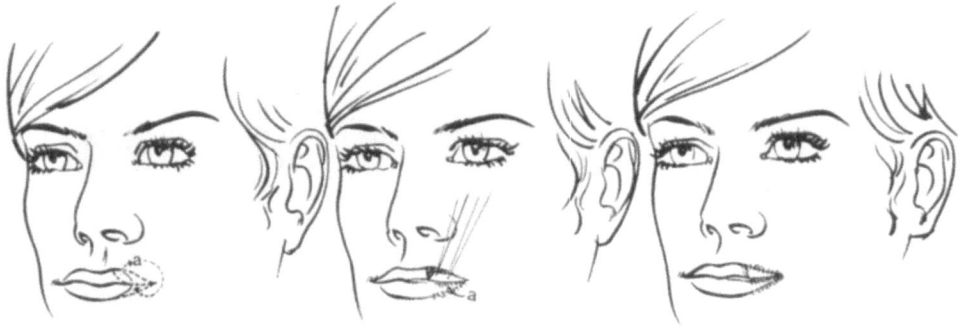

Fig. 43. *Plastic surgery to widen the mouth.* Skin triangles to be excised.

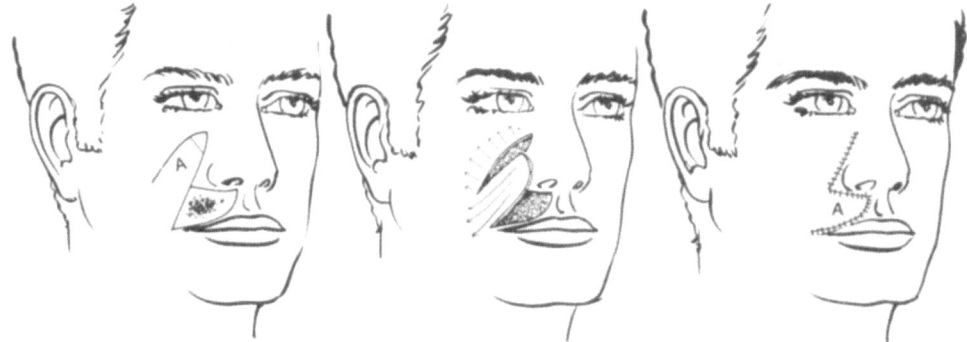

Fig. 44. *Transposition flap technique for upper lip repair.*

functional as well as an aesthetic point of view by using von Burow's advancement flap technique. Two rectangular advancement flaps formed from the cheeks are shifted medially after excision of two Burow's triangles above and below each flap. Wound closure is made by layer (Fig. 45, also called U-flap technique). This procedure is sometimes used on the lower lip as well [79].

3.043 Lower Lip Repair (Spiessl)

This technique consists of three transposition flaps from the nasolabial and cheek region. From this area the incision is continued down over the mandible and sternocleidomastoid muscle to the supraclavicular fossa so that a neck dissection can follow if necessary [182,462]. The nasolabial flap forms the lower lip, the cheek flaps are moved medially, and the last donor site is closed primarily. The lower lip mucous membrane is reconstructed by advancing cheek mucous membrane (Fig. 46.)

3.044 Surgical Therapy for Cheilitis Granulomatosa (Melkersson—Rosenthal Syndrome)

Treatment of choice: transverse submucous triangular excision (Fig. 47 of the granulomatous tissue [97,315]. However, recurrences are to be expected [94].

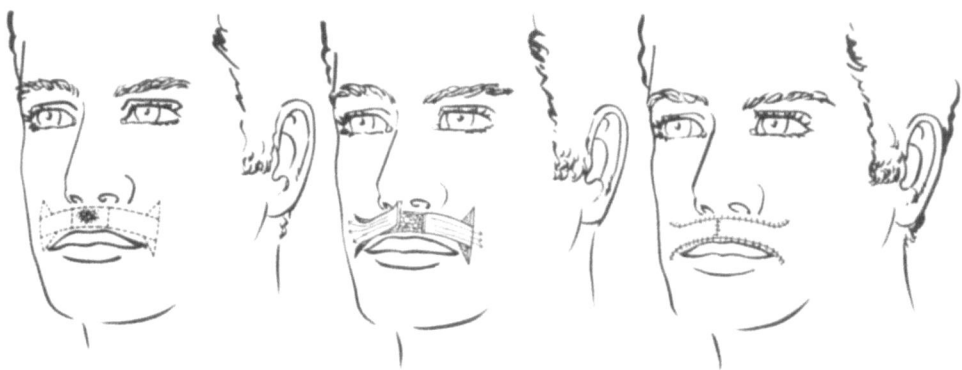

Fig. 45. *Advancement flap technique (von Burow) for upper lip repair.*

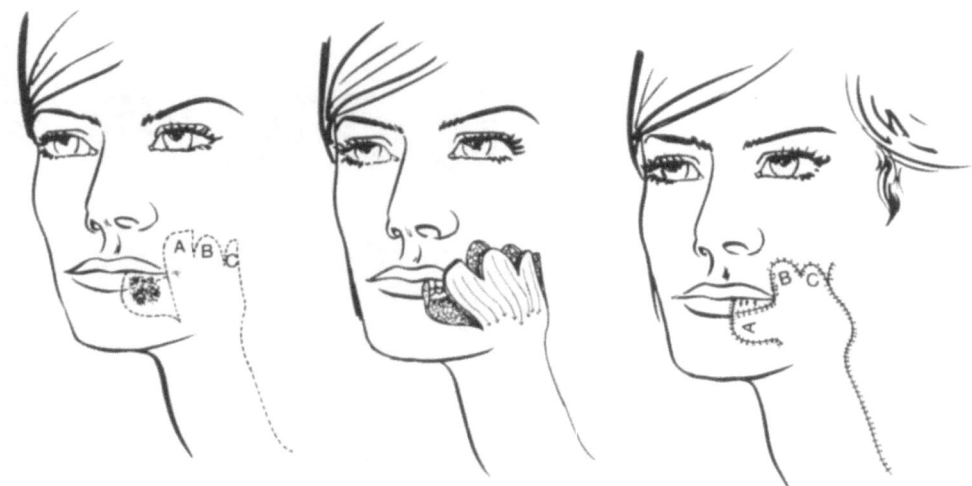

Fig. 46. *Lower lip repair (Spiessl).*

3.045 Correction of Thin Labium

This correction, occasionally desired by female patients, is an uncomplicated operation. After marking the existing labial border and the desired "cupid's bow" shape, local anesthetic is injected and the outlined area excised. The subsequent sutures between skin and labium are best made intracutaneously [293], and the suture line corresponds to the new labial border (cf. Fig. 48).

3.046 Eyelids

In the area of the lower eyelid, the repair of even relatively minor tissue defects can pose difficulties [200,249, 265,270]. Aside from an aesthetically unsatisfactory distortion of the eyelid rims, a primary suture may induce scar eversion and increase the possibility of displacement of the tear ducts with predictably serious consequences [200]. A primary suture of the wound is particularly ill advised in the case of tumors demanding radical removal [317,445]. However, the decision as to the appropriate procedure must be made on a case-to-case basis [33,234,478,479] in order to ensure optimal functional and cosmetic results in each instance [70].

3.047 Advancement Flap Technique (Inner Canthus)

Whether applied caudally or from the superior cranium, this method achieves

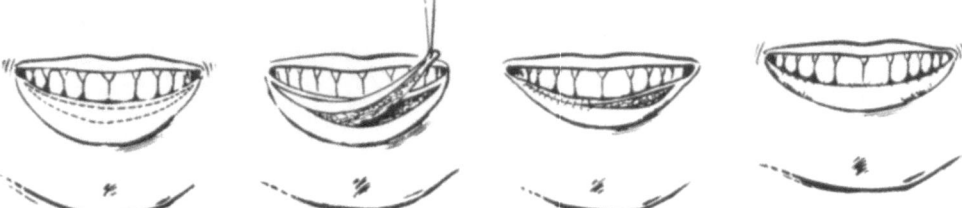

Fig. 47. *Submucous triangular excision for cheilitis granulomatosa.*

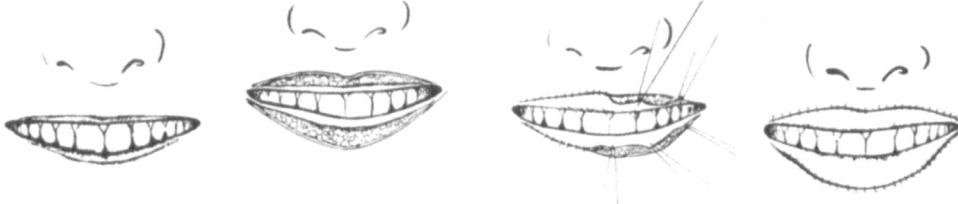

Fig. 48. *Correction of thin labium.*

good results. The technique largely corresponds to that described in Sections 3.023 and 3.024. The additional resultant scars are placed in preformed creases (nasolabial crease and line of the glabella). If there are more extensive defects, it is possible to combine (Figs. 49 and 50) both techniques (Plate 16) [25,213].

3.048 Transposition Flap Technique (Inner Canthus)

After excision of the focus, the surgical defect is closed by a transposition flap from the glabella, and the graft donor site is sutured primarily (Fig. 51). The pedicled forehead flap is, however, aesthetically inferior to the advancement flap [346].

3.049 Advancement—Rotation Flap Technique (Upper Eyelid)

Surgical defects in the medial third of the upper eyelid are with this method

easily repaired from the glabella, where a crescent-shaped skin area is excised to enable a tension-free wound closure (Fig. 52).

3.050 Advancement Flap Technique (Lower Eyelid)

For surgical defects in the medial or lateral third of the lower eyelid or at the outer canthus, a lateral advancement flap is possible following excision of a Burow triangle in the temporal region (Fig. 53).

3.051 Rotation Flap Technique (Imre)

This method is a modified form of the advancement flap technique. After triangular excision of the focus, the incision on the triangle's short side is extended subciliarly in an arc over the temporal region to the preauricular and submental region. The incision should

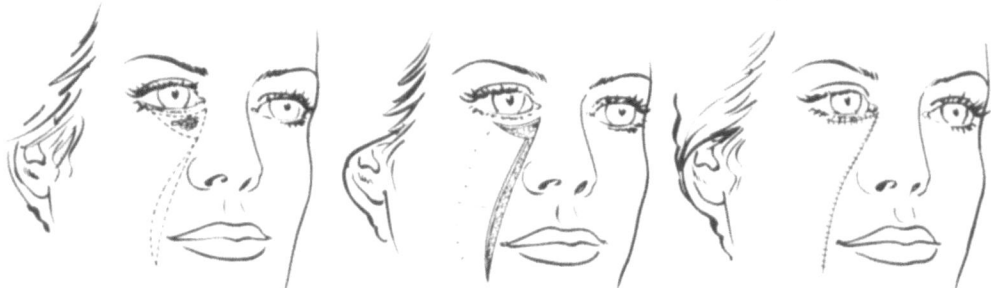

Fig. 49. *Caudal advancement flap technique (inner canthus)* for a median defect of the lower lid.

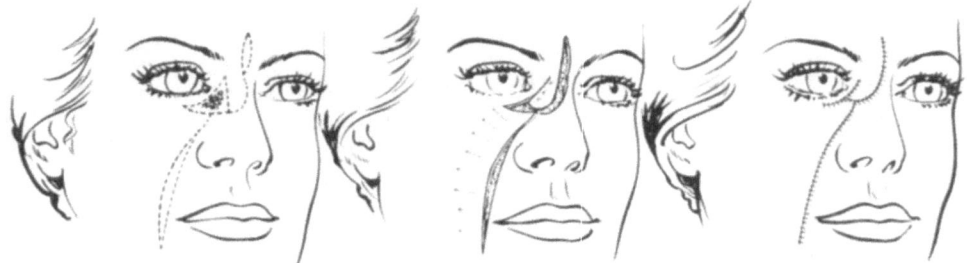

Fig. 50. *Caudal and cranial advancement flap technique (inner canthus).*

follow preformed creases to avoid obvious scars. Then the cheek is mobilized around a central pole [446] and rotated into the surgical defect. The Burow triangle can be made infra- or supraauricularly (Fig. 54, Plate 17). This technique allows replacement of large portions of the lower eyelid, providing the conjunctival mucous membrane remains intact.

3.052 Transposition Flap Technique (Lower Eyelid).

Cosmetically favorable results are achieved in the medial and outer third of the lower eyelid with transposition flaps from the upper eyelid (Plate 18), the supraorbital region or the cheek (Plate 19) [338]. The graft donor site is closed by primary suture. A functionally and aesthetically unsatisfactory shortening of the upper eyelid does not usually occur (Fig. 55). If a tumor involves the conjunctival mucous membrane of the lower eyelid, a transposition flap modified as a composite graft from the upper eyelid can be used [169]. The graft, therefore, contains all layers of the upper eyelid, including tarsus and conjunctival mucous membrane (cf. Fig. 56). Transplanted and autochthonous mucous membranes are connected by submucously tied sutures, and the wound closure is also made layer by layer.

3.053 Correction for Baggy Eyelids (Blepharoplasty).

Correction for baggy eyelids is desired relatively frequently by male and female patients. Our technique of choice [53,67,83,220,386,388,464] is listed by Gebke [155] and Loeb [272].

Warning: Care must be taken not to

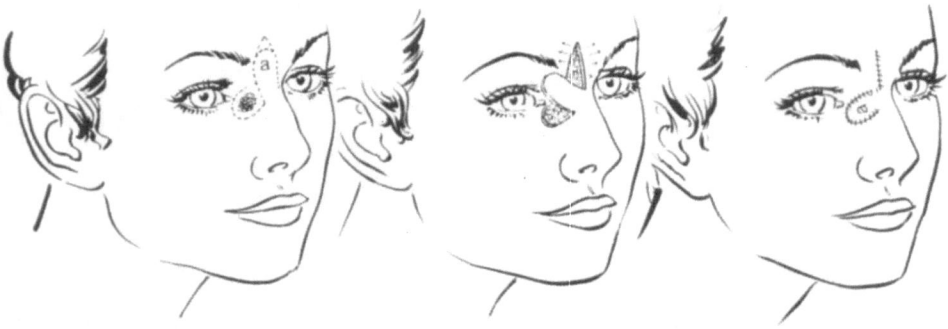

Fig. 51. *Transposition flap technique (inner canthus).*

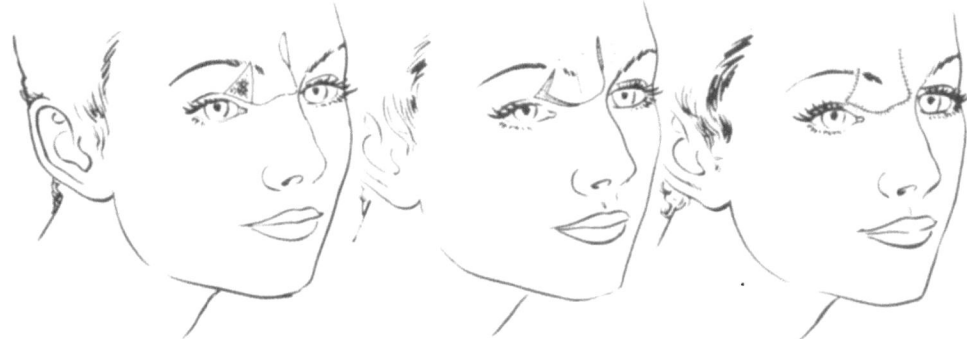

Fig. 52. *Advancement–rotation flap technique (upper eyelid).*

overcorrect [289], because an ectropium may occur on the lower eyelid even if the overcorrection is slight. Because of suturing, milia may occur on the upper eyelid in the scarred area due to displacement of epithelial cells in deeper tissue layers. The occurrence of such cysts is minimized by using very fine, atraumatic suture material [43].

Blepharoplasty on the lower eyelid should basically be performed only by experienced surgeons. Secondary corrections of ectropions after blepharoplasty are not without difficulty and problems. Although extremely rare, cases of blindness in one or both eyes have occurred after blepharoplasty [313]. Possible causes other than retrobulbar hematomas and pressure atrophy of the optic nerve are neuritis and thromboses of the central vein or central artery.

When performing blepharoplasty on the lower eyelid, a subciliary incision is made from the inner to the outer canthus or slightly beyond the eyelashes and then curved slightly down into one of the laugh lines. With dissection scissors, the skin of the lower eyelid is carefully mobilized over a banana-shaped area up to the edge of the orbital bone [155,293,387,388]. In dealing with so-called fat hernias, an incision is subsequently made in the orbital muscle and the exherniated fat tissue resected. Thorough hemostasis is essential. Af-

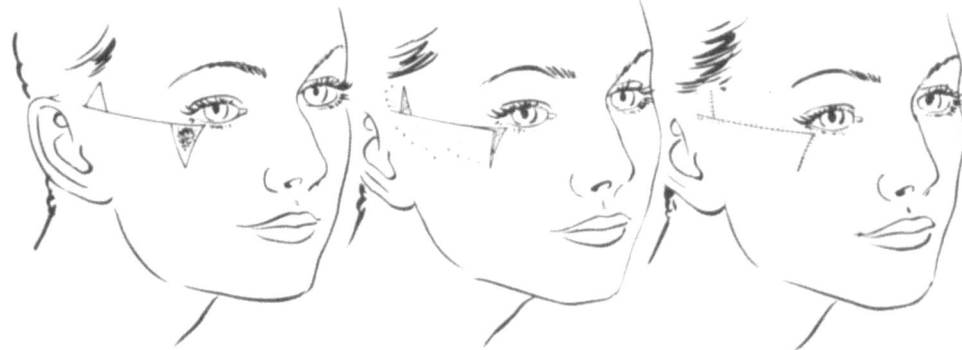

Fig. 53. *Advancement flap technique (lower eyelid).*

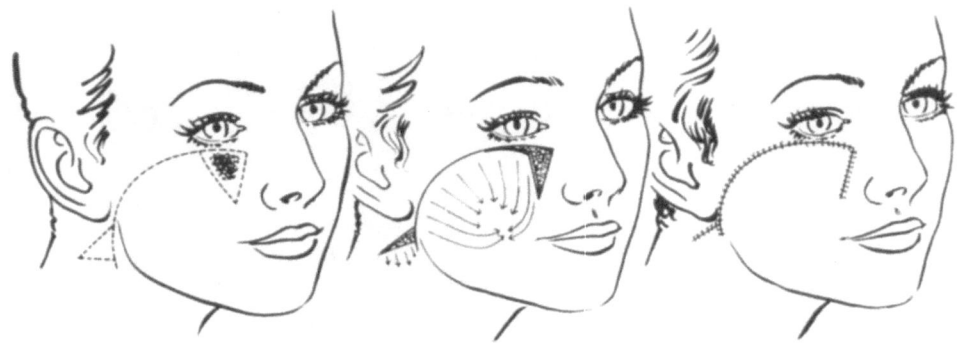

Fig. 54. *Rotation flap technique (Imre)* for defect of the lower eyelid.

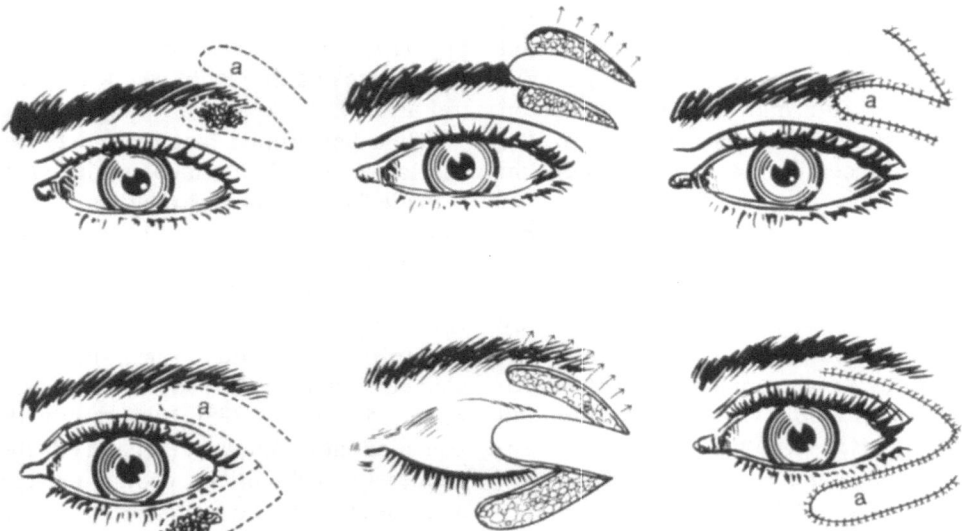

Fig. 55. *Transposition flap technique* (upper eyelid, flap donor site: forehead; lower eyelid, flap donor site: upper eyelid).

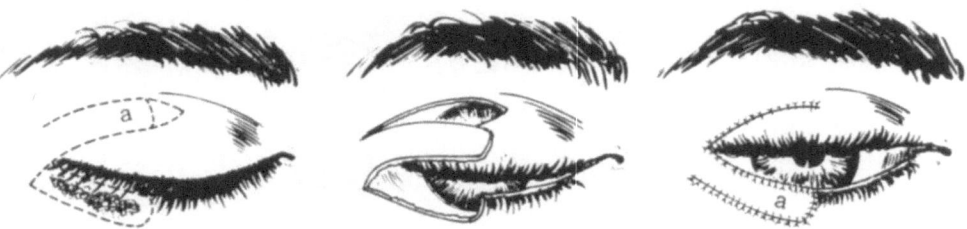

Fig. 56. *Transposition flap technique including conjunctival mucous membrane* (flap donor site: upper eyelid).

terwards the superfluous skin is removed along with a Burow triangle in the area around the outer canthus of the eyelid (for technique cf. Fig. 57, Plate 20).

The blepharoplasty of the upper eyelid is said to be the least problematic and technically the simplest of all cosmetic operations, in marked contrast to that of the lower eyelid [120]. A banana-shaped skin area is usually excised in the region of the palpebral fold. After splitting the orbital muscle, herniated orbital fat tissue is removed, if necessary, followed by thorough hemostasis. Wounds from blepharoplasty are closed either by atraumatic interrupted sutures (Prolene 6–0) or by continuous intracutaneous sutures. In correcting lower eyelids, a fixation suture encompassing the canthal ligament proves expedient.

The W flap (Courtiss, et al., [66]) is an interesting alternative to blepharoplasty of the upper eyelid since superfluous orbital fat tissue is moved with it (Fig. 58).

3.054 Cheeks

In this region the technically more simple free skin grafts are to be avoided as much as possible, for they are functionally as well as aesthetically inferior to a regional flap [266]. Good vascularization of the skin segments to be transplanted facilitates regional flaps in the cheek area [57,58,63,456].

3.055 Advancement Flap Technique

The focus is excised triangularly and the short side of the triangle extended caudally (see Plate 21) or laterally, depending on the operation plan. After it has been undermined, the skin area lying between the tumor excision site and the Burow triangle is advanced into the surgical defect and the defect closed free of tension (Figs. 59 and 60).

3.056 Transposition Flap Technique

This technique is also used on the cheek (Fig. 61). The donor site for the flap is preauricular [442].

3.057 Rotation Flap Technique

This method [cf. 110,352,361] is the same as that used on the lower eyelid, in which the cheek is mobilized around a central pole (Fig. 62, Plate 22).

3.058 Auricle, Pre- and Postauricular Region

If malignancies are involved in the cartilage, surgery is preferred to radiation therapy [38,497].

3.059 Triangular Excision

The simple triangular excision [234,457] is usually sufficient in the case of small neoplasms in the helix area and provides a good cosmetic result [257]. Its advantage is that it can be performed on out-patients under local anesthesia. The adaption of the wound edges is accomplished entirely by interrupted sutures (Fig. 63). Cartilage sutures are not recommended because of the danger of a traumatic ear cartilage necrosis [93,143].

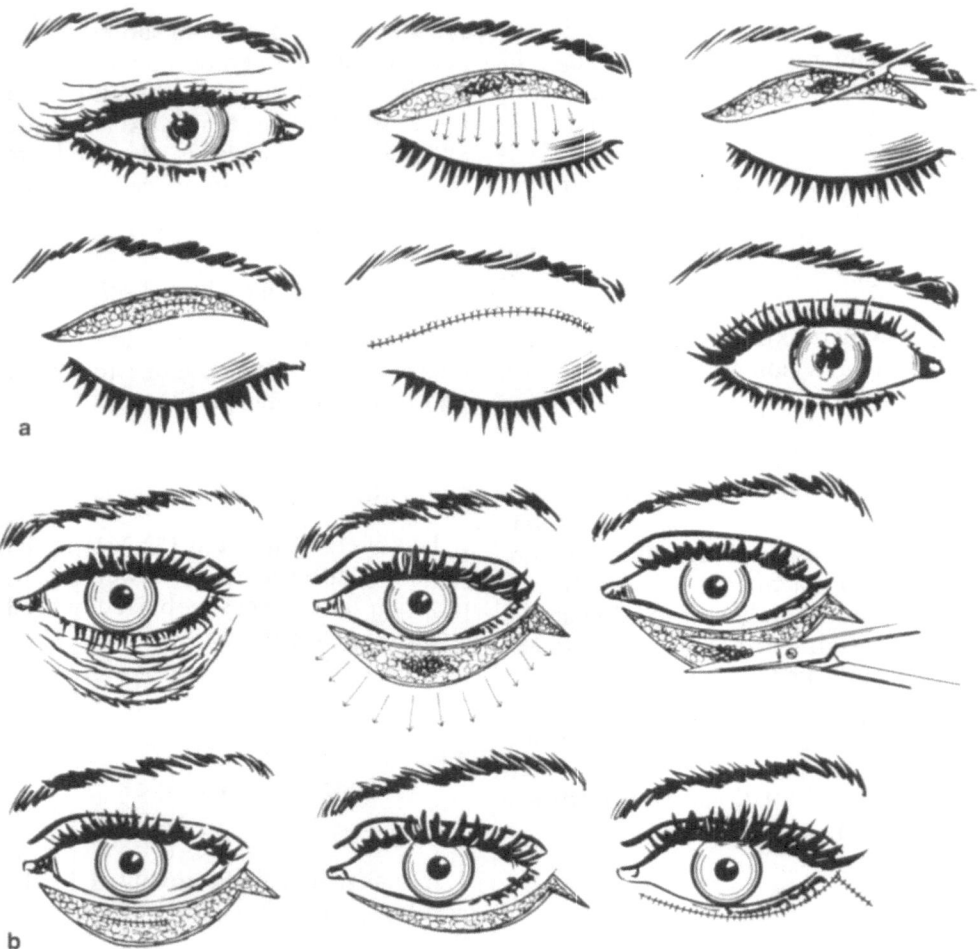

Fig. 57. *Blepharoplasty; **a**,* upper eyelids; ***b**,* lower eyelids.

3.060 Reduction Plasty of the Auricle (Trendelenburg)

If the lateral diameter of an auricle triangular defect is more than a third of the helix after triangular excision, primary sutures of the wound edges result in its ventral folding. Reduction plasty according to Trendelenburg [155,234] is not much more complicated than simple triangular excision and is quite suitable for operations where triangular excision is used. It consists of a triple triangular condrectomy and produces an aesthetically satisfying result (Fig. 64).

3.061 Partial Amputation of the Auricle

If a large part of the auricle must be removed, as much auricle tissue as possible should be retained as the basis for plastic reconstruction or prosthetic supply at a later date.

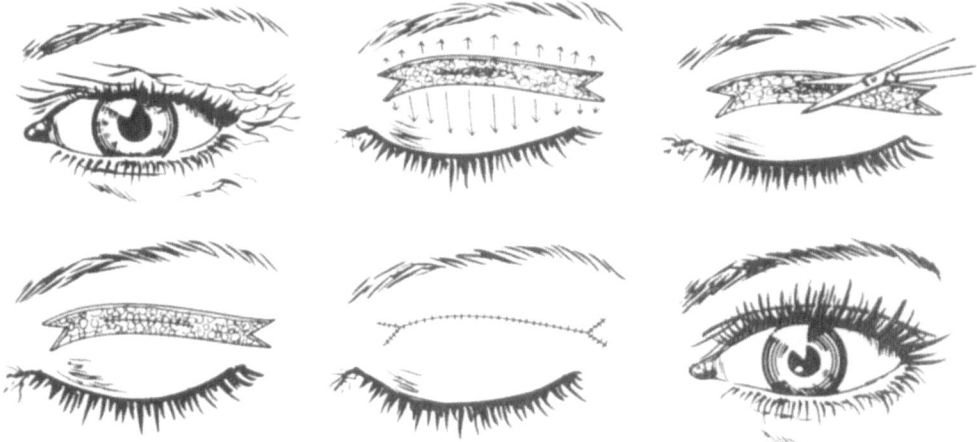

Fig. 58. *Blepharoplasty* (upper eyelid) W-flap technique.

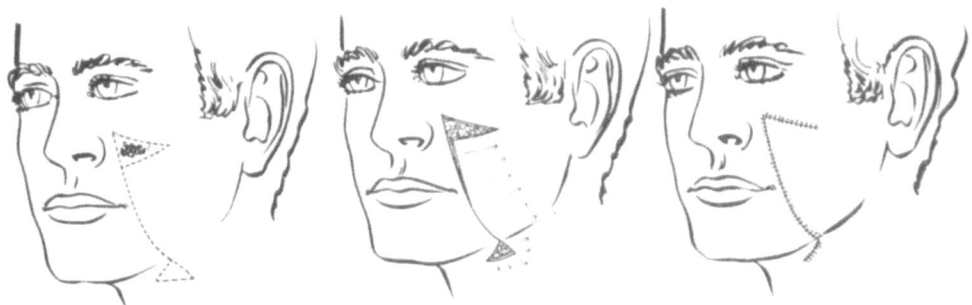

Fig. 59. *Caudal advancement flap technique.*

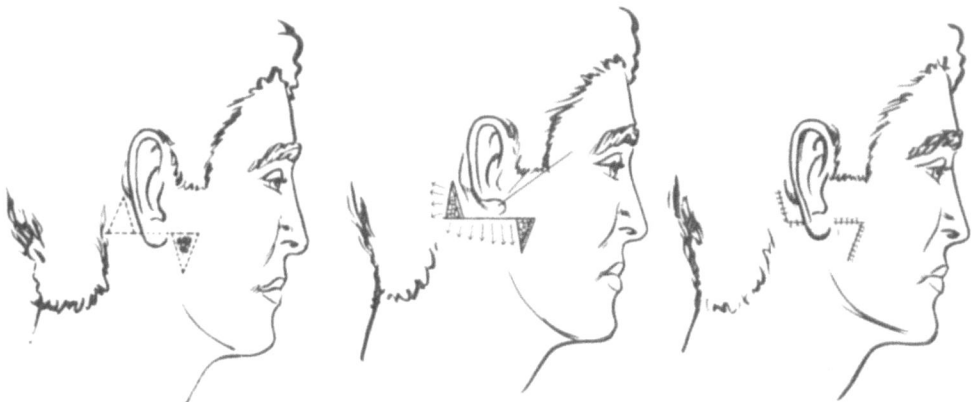

Fig. 60. *Dorsoretroauricular advancement flap technique.*

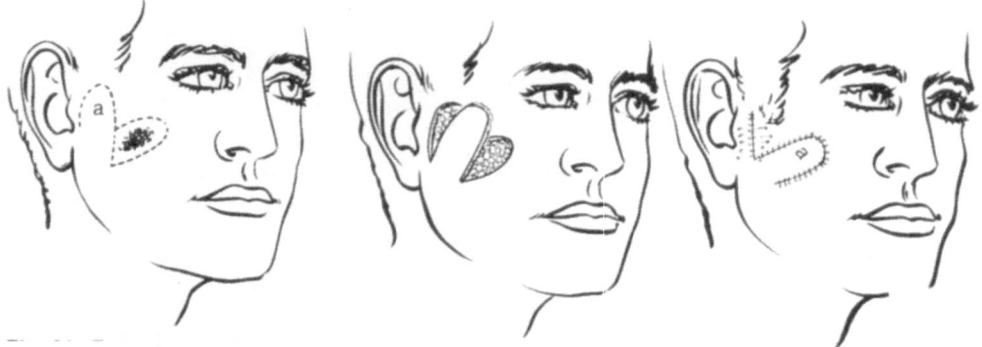

Fig. 61. *Transposition flap technique.*

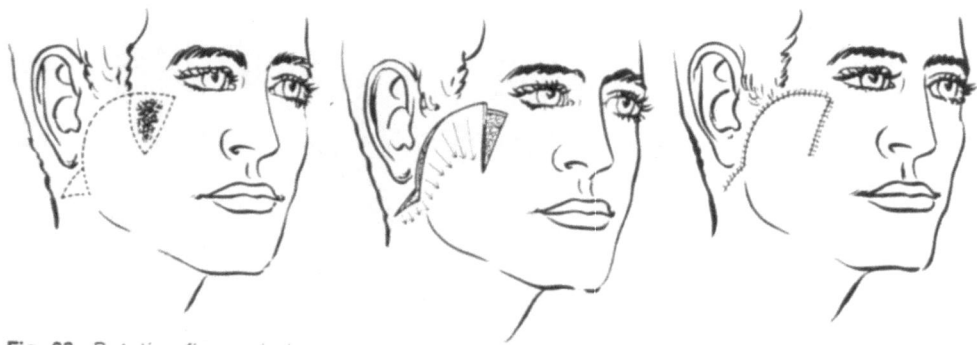

Fig. 62. *Rotation flap technique.*

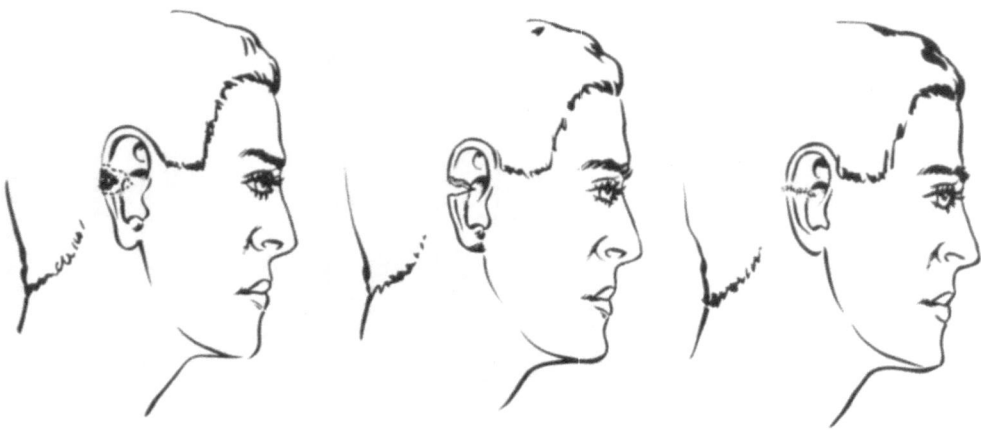

Fig. 63. *Triangular excision—auricle.*

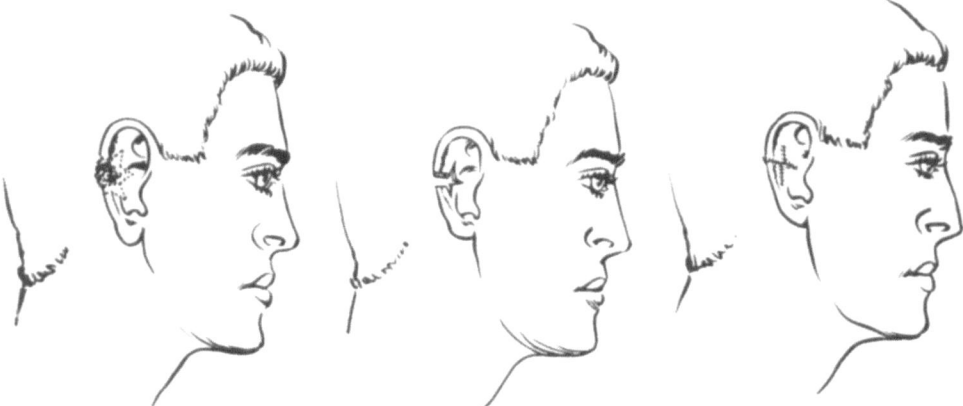

Fig. 64. *Reduction Plasty of the auricle* (Trendelenburg).

3.062 Plastic Reconstruction of the Auricle for Partial Defects

If the upper helix and the ear lobe are retained, a pedicled flap may be affixed with interrupted sutures in the operation defect after undermining the skin retroauricularly. During a second session, the pedicle is cut and used for the reconstruction of the auricle's reverse side. The newly created defect is closed with the aid of a rotation flap from the posterior neck or by a free skin graft.

3.063 Rotation Flap Technique

If the dimensions of a tumor require resection from the retroauricular skin and subcutaneous tissue as well as the auricle's removal, the defect is closed by a rotation flap from the posterior neck (Fig. 65). A wound closure in the region of the mastoid process is possible with this method even if primary suturing or Dehnungsplastik is no longer feasible.

3.064 Transposition Flap Technique

Retro- and preauriculary defects, particularly if the tragus must be re-

moved simultaneously, are repaired by transposition flaps. The pedicles of the flaps may lie supra- or infraauricularly. The flap donor site is closed by primary sutures (Fig. 66, Plates 23–25).

3.065 Advancement Flap Technique

Preauricular tissue defects are closed by a caudal advancement flap, similar to the technique in the cheek area (see Fig. 59). In case of larger wounds, an additional advancement flap from the temporal area should be made in order to achieve a tension-free wound closure. The Burow triangles then lie supra- and infraauricularly (Fig. 67).

3.067 Chin, Throat, and Neck

In the case of nonpenetrating defects of the auricle a subcutaneously pedicled flap from the preauricular area may be used to cover them. The donor site is closed by primary suturing (Fig. 68).

3.067 Chin, Throat, and Neck

Up to average-sized surgical defects in this area can usually be treated by

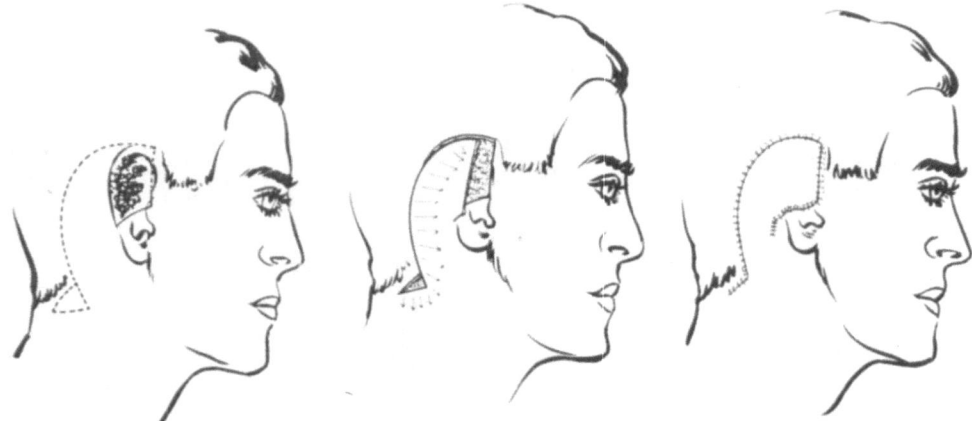

Fig. 65. *Rotation flap technique* for extensive auricle defect.

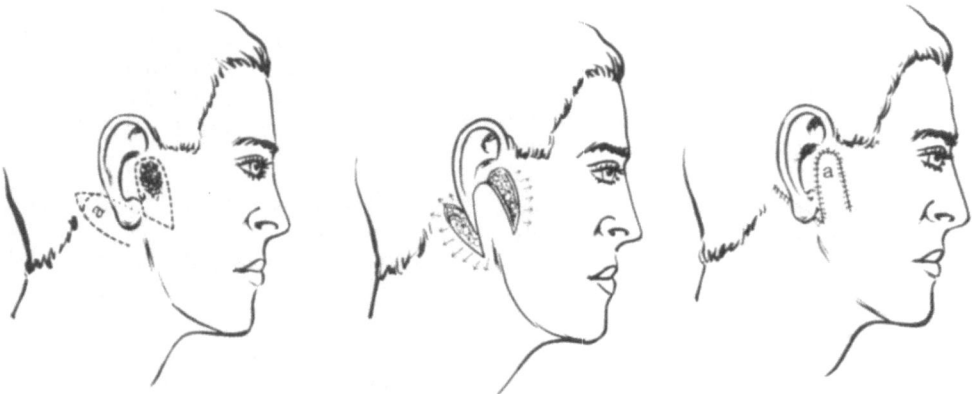

Fig. 66. *Transposition flap technique* for preauricular defect (tragus) (flap donor site: retro-auricular).

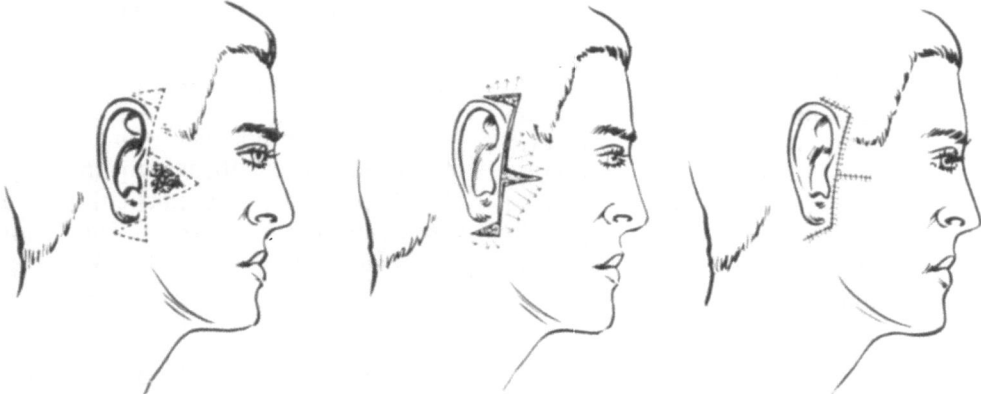

Fig. 67. *Cranial and caudal advancement flap technique* for preauricular defect.

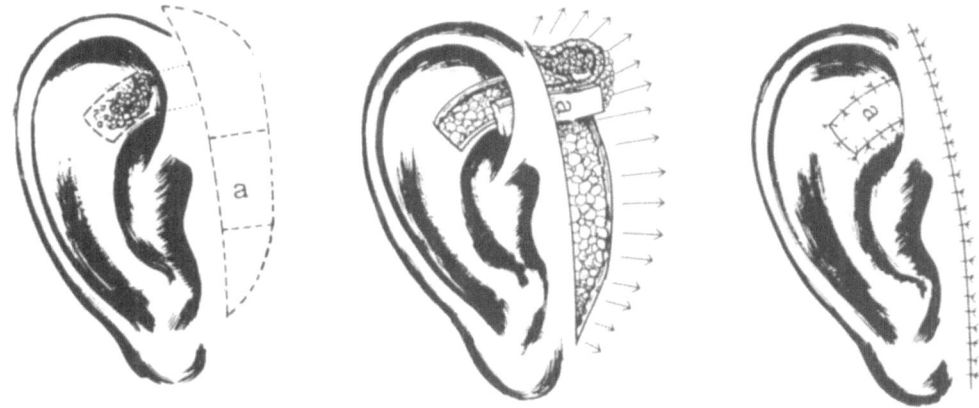

Fig. 68. *Tunnel flap technique* for defects of the auricle.

primary suture or Dehnungsplastik. After undermining of the surrounding skin area, the entire area affected by a dissecting cellulitis of the scalp as well as its subcutaneous tissue is excised elliptically. The surgical defect is then closed with interrupted sutures. Repair with a free autologous skin graft [304] is generally not necessary. More complicated surgical techniques are required only when dealing with larger defects, such as extensive injuries or carcinomas which have arisen on them.

3.068 Advancement Flap Technique

After a half-moon-shaped excision of a focus in the chin area, the resulting

defect is closed by the caudal skin advancement flap technique, Burow triangles having already been made to the right and left supraclavicularly (Fig. 69, also called U-flap technique). Generally, no impairment of facial expression or head mobility results from this technique.

3.069 Rotation Flap Technique (Lateral Chin—Mandibular Area)

After the focus is triangularly excised, the short side of the triangle is lengthened in an arc supraclavicularly and a Burow triangle made on the contralateral side of this incision. The peritomized skin segment is then under-

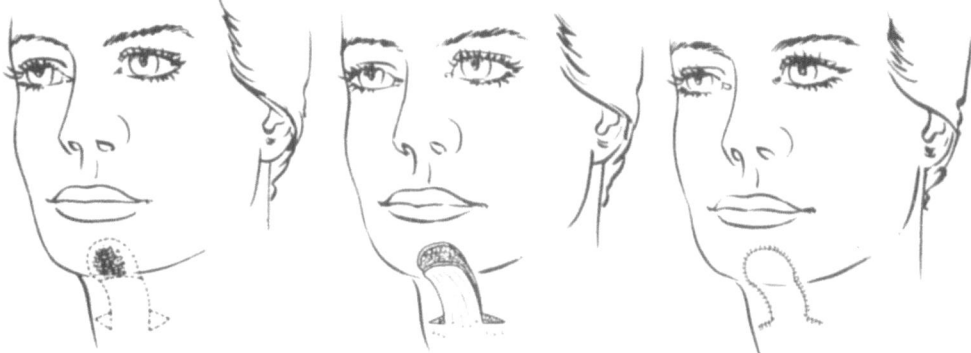

Fig. 69. *Caudal advancement flap technique* for chin defect.

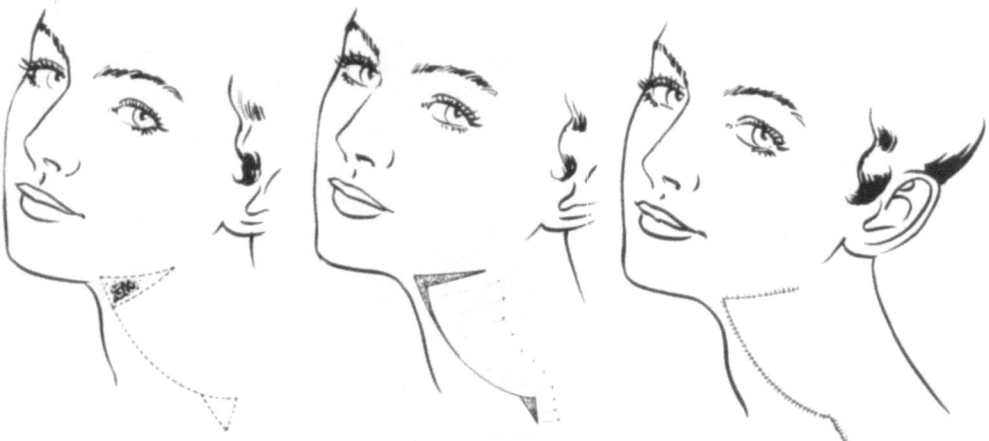

Fig. 70. *Rotation flap technique (lateral chin—mandible defect).*

mined and advanced into the primary surgical defect, which is closed free of tension (Fig. 70).

3.070 Rotation Flap Technique (Throat)

Larger defects in the throat area can be closed by a rotation flap from the thorax (Fig. 71) or by the double rotation flap technique following.

3.071 Double Rotation Flap Technique

The subcutaneously mobilized skin segment is rotated from the chest and the shoulder into the surgical sound (Plate 26).

3.072 Transposition Flap Technique

This technique is especially recommended for those cases where subcu-

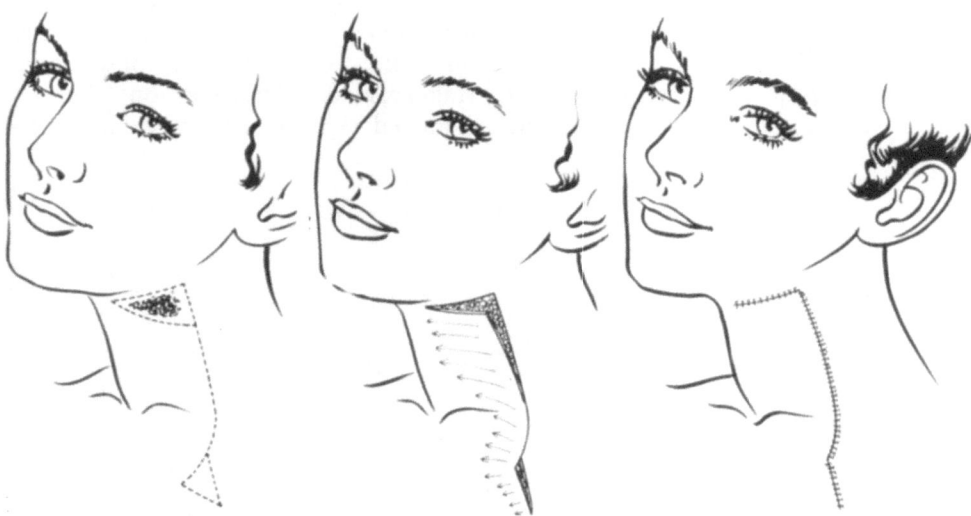

Fig. 71. *Rotation flap technique (throat)*—for larger skin defects.

taneous fat tissue is to be transplanted also (Fig. 72). The donor site is the upper anterior half of the thorax. In most cases it is necessary to partially repair the donor site by free skin grafting [508].

3.073 Trunk

If the defects in this area are so extensive that primary wound closure, even after undermining the wound edges, is impossible [357], the following techniques are applied.

3.074 Transposition Flap Technique

The focus is excised and the defect repaired with a pedicled flap from the surrounding area (Plate 28). If primary suturing of the flap donor site is impossible, it may be repaired by a free skin graft.

3.075 Rotation Flap Technique

The focus is excised triangularly. The incision of the triangle's short side is extended in an arc shape and a Burow triangle is excised on its contralateral side (Fig. 73, Plate 27). After subcutaneously undermining the skin segment lying between the excision site and the Burow triangle, the skin is advanced into the defect and the wound closed free of tension [171].

3.076 Double Rotation Flap Technique

If excision of the focus is made in a circular to ovular shape, two arc-shaped cutaneous incisions are placed at opposite points of the surgical defect. After subcutaneous undermining of the peritomized skin segments, they are rotated counterclockwise into the surgical defect, closing the wound free of tension (Fig. 74). Carcinomas, especially those from scars and radiation injuries and decubital ulcers, which are located in the lumbosacral area are treated according to this principle [185].

3.077 Free Skin Grafting Technique

This procedure is inferior to the local flap on the trunk, both from an aes-

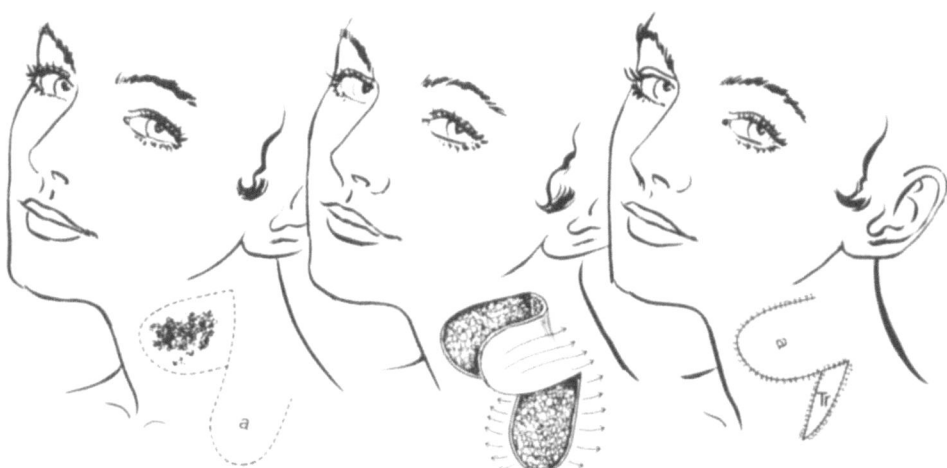

Fig. 72. *Transposition flap technique* for larger skin defect in the area of the thorax. Flap donor site on the thorax partially repaired with free skin graft.

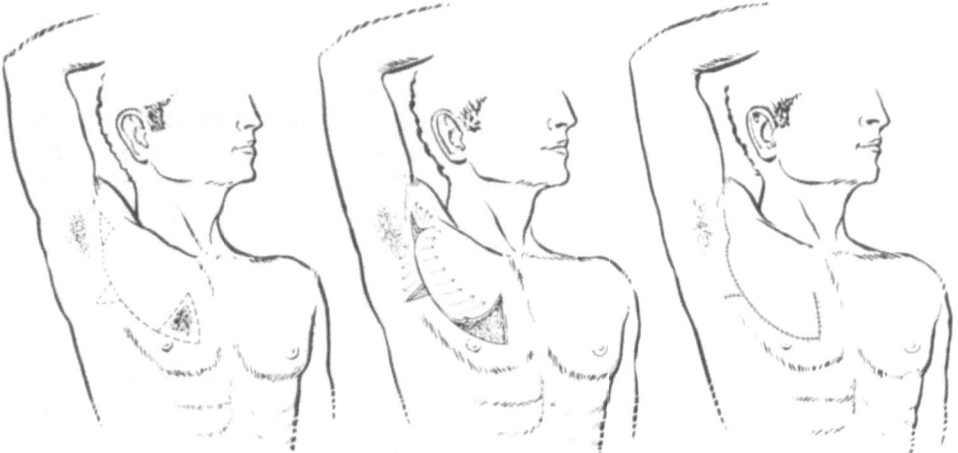

Fig. 73. *Rotation flap technique* in the area of the thorax.

thetic as well as functional point of view. However, the repair of a defect with split-thickness graft may be recommended, if the surgical field must be monitored for recurrencies following tumor removal.

3.078 Rehabilitation of Sagging Abdomen

A correction is occasionally desired for sagging abdominal walls and numerous striation marks. An appropriate technique in terms of a lipectomy was first described in 1910 [237]. However, every plastic rehabilitation of the abdominal wall carries some risk because of the danger of fat emboli. Appropriate prophylactic measures (pharmaceutical) should be considered.

To achieve favorable results with the modified Dehnungsplastik technique (Pitanguy) [372], excise an approximately triangular skin area including the subcutaneous fat tissue. The incision should run in an arc shape from

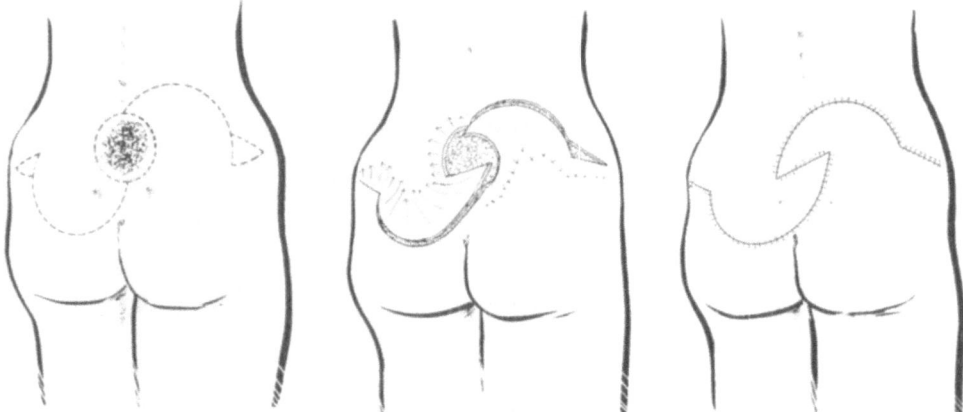

Fig. 74. *Double rotation flap technique* in the sacral area.

the navel to both anterior iliac spines and from there to the symphysis. The remaining abdominal skin is then subcutaneously mobilized as far as the costal arch and the flanks, while the peritomized navel remains in position and is connected by sutures to the abdominal skin, which is already fenestrated and pulled over for this purpose. The wound closure is made primarily with subcutaneous and cutaneous interrupted sutures, but if there is dehiscence of the rectus abdominis muscle, the rectus sheaths must be sutured [172] with nonresorbable suture material, e.g., chromic catgut, 2–0 or Dexon thread. A vertical incision in an abdominal wall rehabilitation is aesthetically less satisfactory [116].

3.079 Axilla

In this region also, small- to average-sized defects may be closed by primary suturing or Dehnungsplastik. The wound closure presents problems if the subcutaneous fat tissue is scarred, for example, after radiation treatment, in this case, plastic repair must be considered.

3.080 Transposition Flap Technique

In this method a skin flap including subcutaneous dorsal fat tissue (lateral edge of the latissimus dorsi muscle) is transposed ventrally into the operation defect (Fig. 75, Plate 28).

3.081 Rotation Flap Technique

The rotation flap is an alternative to the transposition flap method in the area of the axilla (Fig. 76). Especially in cases of chronically recurring hidradenitis suppurativa [236,258,294,407] no longer accessible to conservative therapy, radical excision of the scarred tissue [376,378] and subsequent repair of the defect by a rotation flap effects healing [359].

3.082 Surgical Therapy for Axillary Hyperhidrosis

The varied concentration of the

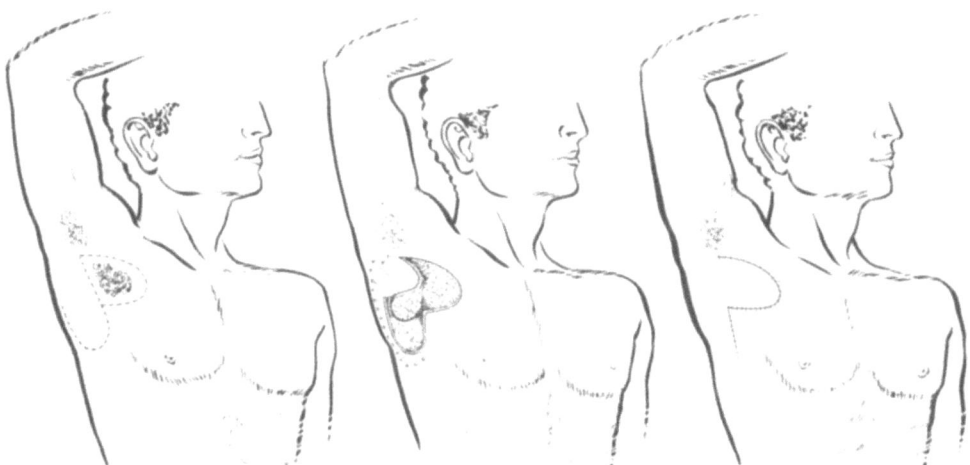

Fig. 75. *Transposition flap technique* in the area of the axilla.

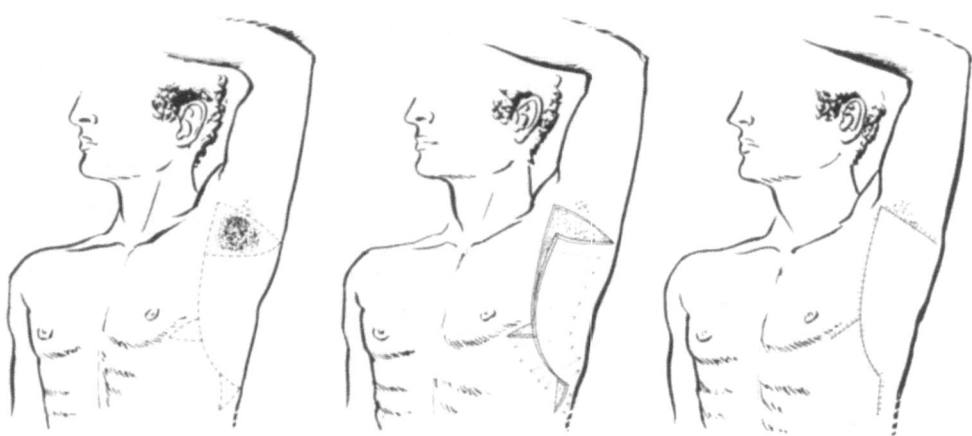

Fig. 76. *Rotation flap technique* in the area of the axilla.

sweat glands is usually ascertained with the observation of spontaneous perspiration after dabbing dry. If this method is insufficient, Minor's sweating test is performed: a solution consisting of iodine, 1.5 g; castor oil, 10.0 ml; alcohol to 100.00 ml is applied with an applicator stick and then powdered with wheat starch. The sweating zone turns bluish black and is marked.

An oval to elliptical excision may be performed either transversely or longitudinally (Fig. 77). The wound closure is made by primary suturing according to the method of Dehnungsplastik [407,492,501].

A recently developed method is subcutaneous hidradenectomy through a small retromammary incision. The sweat glands are removed by a gynecologic curette. Cosmetic results are excellent.

3.083 Male Genital Region

3.084 Dorsal Incision

Dorsal incision is generally recom-
mended for paraphimosis, the most common surgical procedure in the area of the male genitalia. A 1–2 cm (½–¾ in.) incision is made vertically in the direction of the circle of constriction, separating it and enabling a repositioning of the prepuce [412]. The course of the incision afterwards is horizontal.

Warning: Avoid injury to the cavernous bodies.

The wound is closed either by primary sutures or left to heal secondarily. Antibiotic and antiphlogistic follow-up treatment may be necessary in many cases.

3.085 Circumcision

Besides being performed for medical reasons (inflammatory or congenital phimosis), this operation is being increasingly performed today for social-hygienic reasons [78,430]. The outer and inner leaf of the prepuce is excised in the vicinity of the sulcus, after blunt detachment of any synechiae which may be present between the inner leaf of the prepuce and the glans penis. The two leaf stumps are then sutured.

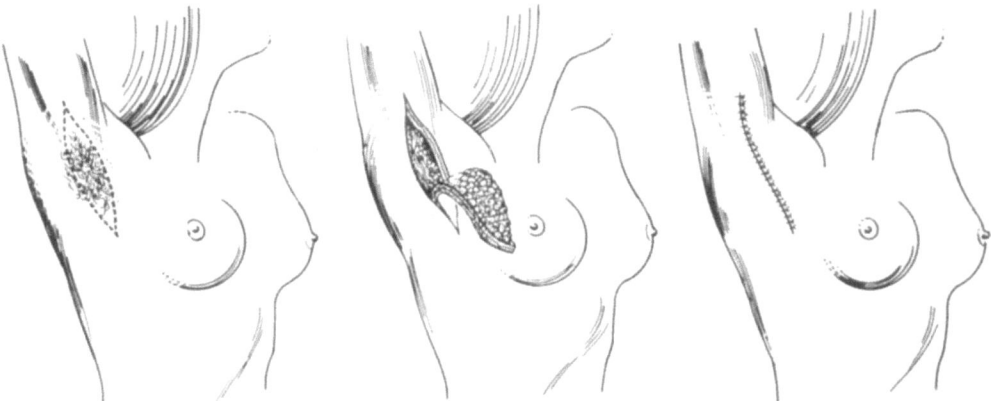

Fig. 77. *Elliptical excision for Hyperlinotrosis axillaris [188a].*

3.086 Phimosis Correction
       (Rebreyoud [385]).

The inner leaf of the prepuce is pulled up tautly and firmly [78] with two Kocher forceps, placed dorsally and ventrally; then the outer leaf is circumcized approximately 5–10 mm above the penile sulcus and dissected from the inner leaf. Then the inner leaf is resected near the sulcus after separation of the frenulum. Suturing should be done with atraumatic catgut sutures between the outer leaf and the stump of the inner leaf of the prepuce so that the stitches are placed in the coronary sulcus (Fig. 78, Plate 29).

3.087 Pedicled Flap Technique
       (Happle)

The operative treatment of precancerous neoplasms of the glans penis (Bowen's disease, erythroplasia of Queyrat) sometimes presents technical difficulties. From a curative as well as aesthetic standpoint, the technique de-

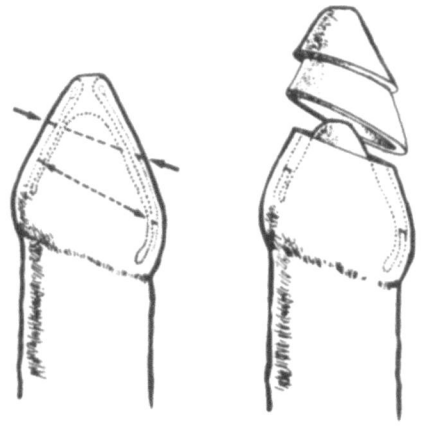
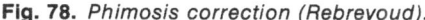
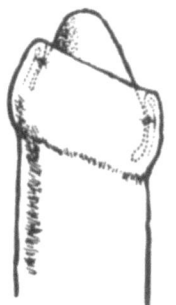
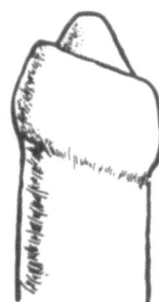

Fig. 78. *Phimosis correction (Rebreyoud).*

scribed by Happle [187] yields favorable results if dealing with circumscribed neoplasms. In this procedure the surgical defect is repaired by means of a pedicled flap from the outer preputial leaf after complete removal of the inner preputial leaf and partial excision of the outer leaf (Fig. 79, Plate 30).

3.088 Amputation of the Penis

If carcinomas of the penis are present, amputation usually cannot be avoided. The radical inguinal lymphadenectomy is performed during one session, even if the presence of enlarged lymph nodes in the inguinal folds cannot be proven by palpation.

It is advisable to perform a lymphangiography prior to surgery in order to exclude iliac and paraaortal metastases. If lymph nodes are suspect, they should also be removed in an appropriately equipped and staffed hospital. If metastases are proven histologically, intensive x-ray therapy is required.

3.089 Repair of a Defect in the Scrotal Area

Since sufficient skin is available, generally a primary suture is not difficult to achieve. In dermatosurgery it is very seldom that a surgical defect must be repaired by free skin grafting.

3.090 Free Skin Grafting Technique

In case of elephantiasis of the penis and scrotum, extensive resection of the indurated cutaneous and hypodermic tissue is required. The surgical defects are repaired by autogenous full-thickness skin grafts [cf. 217, for example] removed with a dermatome. A bladder catheter must be introduced postoperatively and maintained in position for about 8 days.

3.091 Lymphangioplasty (Handley and Zieman [358,570])

This rarely used method is often very successful and without much risk in dealing with a lymphedema [358]. The required subcutaneous implantation of several monofilament nylon threads in the scrotum and the penis shaft is effected by channeling them from a distal to a proximal direction into the subcutis of the lower abdomen. A firm pressure dressing must be applied postoperatively and must be worn approximately 2 months, after which a commercially available elastic bandage suffices (Fig. 80).

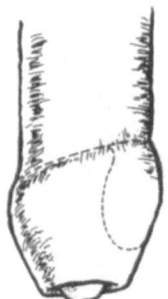 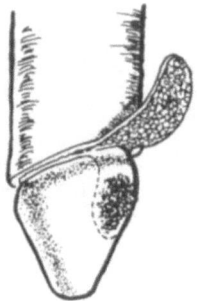 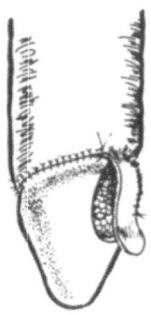 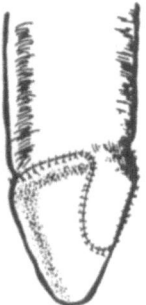

Fig. 79. *Pedicled flap technique (Happle).*

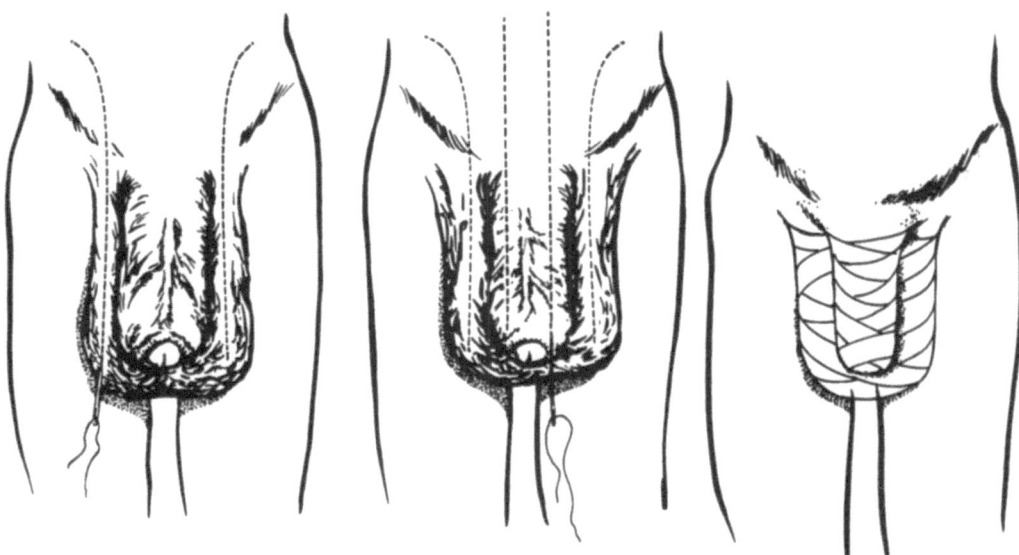

Fig. 80. *Lymphangioplasty (Handley and Zieman)* for elephantiasis of the penis and scrotum.

3.092 Testicular Biopsy

This operation, still important for the diagnosis and prognosis of andrologic diseases, is performed under general or local anesthesia and always on both testicles. If the incision for the biopsy is extended too far caudally or medially, the anatomic features of the testicular arteries increase the risk of vascular injuries with secondary destruction of testicular parenchymae [207]. The assistant's skill is very important, because during the operation he must hold the scrotum between the index and middle fingers of his left hand and, at the same time, gently stretch the scrotal skin tautly over the testicle. The surgeon in this way sees the anterior side of the scrotum without distortion or rotation. After making an approximately 2-cm (¾-in.) incision with the scalpel over the lateral third of the scrotum, the tunica vaginalis of the testicle is separated with the dissecting scissors from the scrotal skin. After splitting the tunica, a self-retaining speculum is inserted and the testicular surface inspected for macroscopic lesions and synechiae. When the least vascularized area of the tunica albuginea has been determined, an incision no longer than 0.5 cm (⅓ in.) is made [408]. Yellowish testicular tissue then exudes and is removed with a small, sharply curved scissors. Closure of the tunica albuginea is made with atraumatic 5–0 catgut; closure of the tunica vaginalis and the scrotal skin, with atraumatic 3–0 to 4–0 catgut.

3.093 Surgery of Varicocele

Surgery of the varicocele, usually performed by the urologist, is rather common in fertilization procedures. It is important to choose one of the techniques which includes high ligation of the genital veins after laparatomy [22,23,208,315,239].

3.094 Female Genital Region

Neoplasms which may still be operated on within dermatosurgery generally require only primary suturing or Dehnungsplastik.

3.095 Vulvectomy

Vulvectomy is occasionally recommended, when treating precancerous neoplasms (kraurosis vulvae) and carcinomas of the external female genitalia. This surgical technique, which in some circumstances makes a displacement of the urethral orifice necessary, should be performed by the gynecologist.

3.096 Extremities

The possibilities for using transposition flaps on the arms and legs are limited for anatomic reasons.

In treating nevi pigmentosi and tattoos, the use of repeated elliptical excisions, closed primarily, each time by Dehnungsplastik, is promising. Treatment of tattoos by high-speed dermabrasion is usually not as successful as desired since the foreign body intrusions are localized in the entire depth of the corium [145].

3.097 Multiple Z Flaps

This technique (cf. Fig. 9) helps alleviate restricted mobility by correcting scar contractures over joints [267,505].

3.098 Transposition Flap Technique

This technique is applied if there is radiogenic injury, e.g., to the subcutaneous tissue, which does not permit a wound closure by primary suture, although this may seem possible initially.

3.099 Free Skin Grafting Technique.

Wound closure is achieved by using free autogenous full-thickness skin grafts [cf. 268] for average-sized surgical defects.

3.100 Surgical Therapy for Leg Ulcers

Leg ulcers due to chronic venous insufficiency comprise a significant portion of dermatosurgery [371,431,459]. A repair of the defect is recommended only after successfully treating the primary bacterial infection, always present in the wound bed, and after eradicating the venous stasis by pressure treatment with, for example, elastic bandages and, in some instances, correctly fitted support hose. These initial treatments are prerequisite to success. Circumcision of the ulcer is not without problems, although it is occasionally recommended, with the aim of inducing proliferation of capillary vessels into the ulcer base and thereby improving the drainage conditions in the chronically inflamed and sclerosed tissue [186]. Ulcers develop in the scars and resist further conservative therapy.

The ulcer repair itself is done either with Reverdin grafts, or sometimes, Wolfe-Krause full-thickness skin grafts or split-thickness skin grafts which may be removed with the dermatome from the contralateral thigh [146,514]. Heterotransplants, such as collagen films, for example, have not proved very helpful as regards duration and result of the therapy.

Reverdin grafts [392] are usually taken from the thigh. With the needle and scalpel held nearly parallel to the skin surface, small patches of skin are pushed up by the needle and separated with the scalpel. The centers of the resultant roundish patches contain epidermis and corium; the edges contain only epidermis. They adhere well to the ulcer base if there are fresh granulations; however, if this does not prove true for individual patches, the procedure is repeated until a complete repair is effected. A good pressure dressing is as important for lasting success as continued treatment of the underlying venous insufficiency. The procedure itself is very simple and the resulting scars withstand pressure well, yet are often cosmetically undesirable. This also applies especially to the multiple circular graft donor sites which spontaneously reepithelize from the wound edges.

This disadvantage of unsightly scarring must be considered, especially when treating younger women. However, the use of punch grafts [146] minimizes these negative results. In this procedure, very small, full-thickness skin (Wolfe-Krause) patches are taken under local anesthesia with the rotating electric punch from a suitable and cosmetically irrelevant skin area (often from the thigh) [248]. Donor sites are closed by interrupted sutures and covered, as in the case of skin-biopsy sites, by a common bandage with antimicrobial powder, producing relatively unnoticeable scars. The subcutis is separated from the punch cylinders with the scalpel and the skin grafts inserted like cobble stones into the ulcer. The site to be repaired is covered with fatty tulle, as is done with patch grafts. A pressure dressing is applied, usually with a foam rubber compress which has been cut to fit, and is not changed for 5 days. Because of the risk of a thrombosis, pa-

tients should not be ambulatory for 2 or 3 days after the operation, and then usually with a correctly applied elastic bandage. This procedure is especially suitable for small ulcers since it is repeatable and may be performed in the office.

The repair of ulcers with a split-thickness graft is somewhat more complicated. The material is taken from the thigh, "thinly" (25%) to "thickly" (75% of the local cutis cover) with the dermatome, depending on requirement of receiver site [146]. The donor site heals with fatty dressings, forming slight to barely noticeable scars. If the cosmetic results are important, the patient must be warned that protection from sunlight is necessary during the first year in order to avoid pigmentation. The split-thickness grafts are fitted into the ulcer and usually affixed by sutures and pressure dressing. Individual incisions are made in larger grafts to facilitate drainage.

The mesh graft represents a new technique. Split-thickness skin is perforated with cross-hatched incisions and is then pulled apart as a fenestrated flap similar to a net. This allows the repair of large wound areas with a small amount of split-thickness material, for example, when dealing with burns.

Another form of split-thickness skin grafting especially suited to the leg ulcer is what is termed "chessboard" graft [146]. A small split-thickness flap is cut in several pieces and transplanted. This compromise between Reverdin's or the punch graft technique and split-thickness skin repair offers good results even for wound areas with heavy drainage.

The Cockett operation is recommended for treating therapy refractory ulcers in the medial malleolar area

[186]. The posterior archuate vein is exposed with a longitudinal incision and extirpated after ligating Cockett's veins. The ulcer area is dissected up to the fascia and the responsible defective communicating vein is ligated and cut. The ulcer is then covered by free skin grafting.

3.101 Hands and Feet

In this area, there are even more anatomic and functional limitations posed to wound closure by primary suture or Dehnungsplastik than on the arms and legs. Prior to surgery the extent of the operation is carefully estimated and the hand surgeon consulted if in doubt.

3.102 Free Skin Grafting Technique

Method of choice: free autogenous full-thickness skin grafts [142]. Full-thickness skin grafts possess important advantages over split-thickness skin grafts. Besides their more favorable cosmetic results [389], they also show less tendency to shrinkage, an improved sensibility, and increased capacity of the graft to bear stress (cf. Plate 31).

3.103 Transposition Flap Technique

If a surgical defect occurs over an interphalangeal joint, the defect is repaired by a transposition flap from the lateral side of the phalange [277]. The donor site is either sutured primarily (Plate 32) or covered by a free skin graft.

3.104 VY-Flap Technique

In some specific cases, e.g., in the posterior hand area, the VY flap [142] is applied successfully on small operation defects.

3.105 Multiple Z-Flap Technique

This method is also applied successfully in treating contracture over finger joints caused by scarring.

3.106 Dermabrasion

Dermabrasion of mycotically involved nails is necessary before successful topical application of antimycotic drugs. Local anesthesia is generally not necessary.

3.107 Nail Extraction

After being loosened under conduction anesthesia with special extraction forceps, the nail can be removed effortlessly.

3.108 Nail Extraction Combined with Triangular Excision

In treating ingrown toenails, recurrences cannot be avoided if nail extraction alone is performed. Therefore, after nail extraction, excision with the scalpel of any surplus granulations possibly present is recommended. Afterwards, the lateral quarter of the nail matrix is removed prophylactically by trangular excision.

Warning: Pay attention to the distal interphalangeal joint!

3.109 Triangular Excision (Emmet)

Only the affected medial or lateral third of the nail, including the nail matrix, is removed by triangular excision. The remaining nail is left intact (cf. 158).

Bibliography

1. Achten, G., Van Oost, A., Ledoux-Corbusier, M.: 5-Fluorouracil (5-Fu) ointment in the treatment of basal cell epithelioma. Histological control over a long duration. Dermatologica (Basel) **140**, Suppl. 1, 59-64 (1970).
2. Allington, H.V., Allington, J.H.: Eyelid tumours. Arch. Derm. (Chic.) **97**, 50-65 (1968).
3. Allington, H.V., Allington, R.R.: Cryosurgery. In: Skin Surgery (ed. E. Epstein), 2nd ed., pp. 299-307. Philadelphia: Lea & Febiger 1962.
4. Anderson, R., Kurtay, M.: Reconstruction of the corner of the mouth. Plast. Reconstr. Surg. **47**, 463-464 (1971).
5. Andina, F.: Plastic surgery of head and neck tumours. International Congress Series No. 98. Amsterdam: Excerpta Medica Foundation 1965.
6. Andina, F: Die freien Hauttransplantationen. Berlin-Heidelberg-New York: Springer 1970.
7. Andrews, E.B.: Repair of lower lip defects by the Hagedorn rectangular flap method. Plast. Reconstr. Surg. **34**, 27(1964).
8. Andrews, E.B.: Island flaps in facial reconstruction. Plast. Reconstr. Surg. *44*, 49–51 (1969).
9. Argamaso, R.V.: V-Y-S-plasty for closure of a round defect. Plast. Reconstr. Surg. **53**, 99–101 (1974).
10. Antoine, L: In: Plastische Chirurgie und Kosmetik (eds. H.v. Seemen, L. Antoine). Vienna-Innsbruck: Urban & Schwarzenberg 1958.
11. Auberger, H.G.: Praktische Lokalanaesthesie, 3rd ed. Stuttgart: G. Thieme 1974.
12. Aufricht, G.: Chirurgische Korrektur des alternden Gesichts. In: K. Schuchardt: Fortschritte der Kiefer- und Gesichtschirurgie, Vol. VII. Stuttgart: Thieme 1961.
13. Ayres, S.: Superficial chemosurgery. In: Skin Surgery, (ed. E. Epstein), 2nd ed., pp. 268–298. Philadelphia: Lea and Febiger 1962.
14. Ayres, S., Ayres, S: Endothermy and Elektrocoagulation. In: Skin Surgery (ed. E. Epstein), 2nd ed., pp. 189–201. Philadelphia: Lea & Febiger 1962.
15. Bandmann, H.J.: Aufgaben des Dermatologen bei der Früherkennung des Krebses. Die Treffsicherheit einer fachärztlich gestellten klinischen Diagnose. In: Fortschr. prakt. Derm. Venerol. (eds. O. Braun-Falco, D. Petzoldt), Vol. 7, pp. 30–35. Berlin-Heidelberg-New York: Springer 1973.
16. Barton, M., Spira, M., Hardy, S.B.: An improved method for "V" excision of the lip combined with vermilionectomie. Plast. Reconstr. Surg. **33**, 471–473 (1964).
17. Baumgartl, E. Kremer, K., Schreiber, H.W. (eds.): Spezielle Chirurgie für die Praxis, Vol. I, Part 1. Stuttgart: Thieme 1973.
18. Baumgartner, P.: Schönheit und Verjüngung durch kosmetische Chirurgie? Stuttgart: Thieme 1972.
19. Belisario, J.C.: Chemotherapie des Hautkrebses. Hautarzt **14**, 438–443 (1963).
20. Bell, R.C.: The use of skin grafts. In: Monographs on Plastic Surgery, Vol. I. London-New York-Toronto: Oxford Univ. Press 1973.
21. Bernard, C.: Cancer de la lèvre inférieure; restauration á l'aide de lambeux quadrilataires-latereaux querison. Scalpel (Liège) **5**, 162–165 (1851-1853).
22. Bernardi, R.: Varicocele. Resultados obtenidos en 500 casos con un procedimento personal. Rev. argent. Urol. **26**, 152–168 (1957).
23. Bernardi, R.: Varicocele. The results obtained in 500 cases with a personal procedure. J. Amer. Med. Assoc. **61,** 57 (1958).

24. Bethmann, W., Zoltán, J.: Operationsmethoden der plastischen Chirurgie. Jena: VEB Gustav Fischer 1968.
25. Blaskovics, L., Kreiker, A.: Eingriffe am Auge. Stuttgart: Enke 1959.
26. Bode, H.G.: Strahlentherapie der Hautkrankheiten. In: E. Riecke: Lehrbuch der Haut- und Geschlechtskrankheiten, pp. 800–828. Stuttgart: G. Fischer 1962.
27. Bode, H.G., Theismann, H., Renzishausen, H., Volkmann, J.: Strahlenreaktion und peripherer Kreislauf. Derm. Wschr. 121, 218–222 (1950).
28. Boette, G.: Über Röntgenkrebse und Röntgenbestrahlung im Halsbereich. Aesthet. Med. 9, 57–61 (1960).
29. Böttger, H.: Geschwulstoperation: Prothetische und epithetische Maßnahmen. Diagnostik 6, 764–766 (1973).
30. Borges, A.F., Alexander, J.E.: Relaxed and skin tension lines, Z-plastics on scars and friform excisions of lesions. Brit. J. Plast. Surg. 15, 242 (1962).
31. Borges, F.A., Alexander, J.E., Block,L.I.: Z-Plasty treatment of unesthetic scars. Eye, Ear, Nose Throat Mon. 44, 39–44 (1965).
32. Borghouts, J.M.H.: Surgical treatment of basal cell carcinoma and squamous cell carcinoma of the skin. Arch. Chir. Neerl. 16, 19–30 (1964).
33. Bostwick, F., Vasconez, L.O., Furkiewicz, M.F.: Basal cell carcinoma of the medial canthal area. Plast. Reconstr. Surg. 55, 667–676 (1975).
34. Bowers, D.G.: Double cross-lip flaps for lower lip reconstruction. Plast. Reconstr. Surg. 47, 209–214 (1971).
35. Brabetz, V.: Schädigungen durch Kosmetik. Z. Hautkr. 8, 156–163 (1950).
36. Braun-Falco, O., Burg, G.: Cytostatica und Immunsuppressiva in der Dermatologie. Hautarzt 21, 391–397 (1970).
37. Braun-Falco, O.: Maligne epitheliale Tumoren im Geisichtsbereich. In: Plastische Chirurgie des Kopf-und Halsbereiches und der weiblichen Brust (ed. H. Bohmert). Stuttgart: Thieme 1975.
38. Braun-Falco, O., Lukacs, S., Goldschmidt, H.: Dermatoradiotherapy. New York-Heidelberg-Berlin: Springer 1976.
39. Brehm, K., Hundeiker, M.: Eine Methode zur Behandlung von Praecancerosen der Haut. Z. Hautkr. 49 (1974).
40. Breslow, A.: Tumor thickness, level of invasion and node dissection in stage I cutaneous melanoma. Ann. Surg. 182, 572–575 (1975).
41. Brown, J.B., McDowell, F.: Plastic Surgery of the Nose, St. Louis: C.V.Mosby 1951.
42. Brown, J.B., McDowell, F.: Skin Grafting. Philadelphia: Lippincott 1958.
43. Bruck, H.G.: Chirurgisch-kosmetische Indikationen in Jugend und Alter. Aesthet. Med. 17, 245–250 (1968).
44. Bruns, V.von: Die chirurgische Pathologie und Therapie des Kau- und Geschmacksorgans. In: Handbuch der praktischen Chirurgie (ed. V. von Bruns), Vol. I, part 1: Die äußeren Weichteile. Tübingen: Laupp 1859.
45. Bryant, J.D.: Operative Surgery. 4th ed., Vol. I. New York: D. Appleton & Comp. 1906.
46. Buff, H.U.: Hautplastiken. Indikation und Technik. Stuttgart: Thieme 1952.
47. Burg, G. Mikroskopisch kontrollierte (histographische) Chirurgie. In: Dermatochirurgie in Klinik und Praxis (ed. B. Konz, G. Burg), pp. 72–82. Berlin-Heidelberg-New York: Springer 1977.
48. Burket, J.M.: Vermilionectomy for lower lip leukoplakia. Arch. Dermatol. 95, 397–399 (1967).
49. Burow, A.v.: Beschreibung einer neuen Transplantationsmethode (Methode der seitlichen Dreiecke) zum Wiederersatz verlorengegangener Teile des Gesichts. Berlin 1856 (zit. nach v. Bruns).
50. Cameron, R.R., Latham, W.D., Dowling, J.A.: Reconstructions of the nose and upper lip with nasolabial flaps. Plast. Reconstr. Surg. 52, 145–150 (1973).
51. Caro, M.R.: The biopsy. In: Skin Surgery (ed. E. Epstein), 2nd ed., pp. 185–188. Philadelphia: Lea & Febiger 1962.
52. Castenares, S.: Blepharoplasty for herniated intraorbital fat teratomical basis for a new approach. Plast. Reconstr. Surg. 8, 46–58 (1951).
53. Christ, W.: Sekundäre plastische Deckung ausgedehnter infizierter Hautdefekte. Aesthet. Med. 10, 275–278 (1961).
54. Clark, W.H., From, L., Bernardino, E.A., Mihm, M.C.: The histogenesis and biologic behavior of primary human malignant melanomas of the skin. Cancer Res. 29, 705–726 (1969).
55. Cohney, C.: Reconstruction de la livre inférieure après excision chirurgicale pour cancer. Ann. Chir. Plast. (Paris) 8, 105 (1963).
56. Conley, J.: Management of malignant tumours of the scalp. Ann.N.Y. Acad. Sci, 114, 976–984 (1964).
57. Conley, J., Dickinson, J.T.: Plastic and re-

constructive surgery. Proceedings of the first international symposium, Vols.I,II. Stuttgart: Thieme 1972.

58. Conley, J.: Regional Flaps of the Head and Neck. Stuttgart: G. Thieme 1976.

59. Conrad, F.G.: Treatment of malignant melanoma. Wide excision vs. lymphadenectomy. Arch. Surg. **104**, 587–593 (1972).

60. Converse, J.M.: Plastic surgery and transplantation of skin. In: Skin Surgery (ed. E. Epstein), 2nd ed., pp. 92–126. Philadelphia: Lea & Febiger 1962.

61. Converse, J.M.: Reconstructive Plastic Surgery. Principles and Procedure in Correction, Reconstruction and Transplantation, Vols.I,II. Philadelphia-London: W.B. Saunders 1964.

62. Converse, J.M., Wood-Smith, D.: Deformities of the lips and cheeks. In: Converse, J.M., Reconstructive Plastic Surgery. Philadelphia and London: W.B. Saunders 1964.

63. Conway, H., Seddar, J.: Report of the loss of pigment in full thickness anaplastic skin grafts in the mouse. Plast. Reconstr. Surg. **18**, 30–36 (1956).

64. Corso, P.F.: The use of regional flaps for reconstructive procedures of the head and neck area including oropharyngostomas. In: Conley, J., Dickinson, J.T.: Plastic and Reconstructive Surgery of the Face and Neck, Vol. II: Rehabilitation Surgery. Stuttgart: Thieme 1972.

65. Cosman, B., Niklison, J.: Reconstruction of the facial muscles, lips, and cheeks. In: Grabb, W.C., Smith, J.W., Plastic Surgery. A Concise Guide to Clinical Practice. London: J. & A. Churchill 1968.

66. Courtiss, E.H., Webster, R.C., White, M.F.: Use of double W-plasty in upper blepharo-plasty. Plast. Reconstr. Surg. **53**, 25–28 (1974).

67. Cronin, T.D.: Marginal incision for upper blepharoplasty. Plast. Reconstr. Surg. **49**, 14–17 (1972).

68. Curri, S.B., Manzoli, U., Tischendorf, F.: Die Fingerbeerenbiopsie. Klin. Wochenschr. **44**, 584–590 (1966).

69. Davis, N.C., McLeod, G.R.: The surgery of primary melanoma. Problems and practice. Med. J. Aust. **1972/2**, 778–781 (1972.

70. Dayal, Y., Hill, J.C.: Surgical treatment of tumors of the eyelids. Can. Med. Assoc. J. **93**, 997–1003 (1965).

71. Denecke, H.J.: Die Carcinom-Chirurgie des alternden Antlitzes. Aesthet. Med. **13**, 57–59 (1967).

72. Denecke, H.J.: Plastische Chirurgie bei An-
omalien, Defekten und 'Narben. Aesthet. Med. **18**, 17–24 (1969).

73. Denecke, H.J., Meyer, R.: Plastische Operationen an Kopf und Hals. Vol. I: Korrgierende und rekonstruktive Nasenplastik. Berlin-Göttingen-Heidelberg-New York: Springer 1964. ·

74. Denecke, H.J.: Kefektdeckung nach Operationen von Nasentumoren. Chir. plastica (Berl.) **3**, 219–221 (1967).

75. Dieffenbach, J.F.: Operative Chirurgie, Vol. I. Leipzig: F.A. Brockhaus 1845.

76. Dieffenbach, J.F.: Surgical observations on the restoration of the nose and on the removal of polypi and other tumours from the nostrils (from the German, with the history and physiology of rhinoplastic operations, notes, and additional cases by John Stevenson Buchnan). London: Higley 1833.

77. Dietz, O.: Beitrag zur Technik der Beschneidung. Hautarzt **4**, 172–174 (1954).

78. Dietz, O.: Erfahrungsbericht über 2800 Zirkumzisionen (eine sexualhygienische Betrachtung). Dermatol. Monatschr. **156**, 1029–1034 (1970).

79. Dirvana, S.: Die chirurgische Behandlung des Unterlippenkarzinoms. Berl. Med. **16**, 567–570 (1965).

80. Drepper, H., Ehring, F.: Patientendemonstration Nr. 23. Verhandl. Dtsch. Dermat. Ges., 27. Tagung, Freiburg, 29.9.-3.10. 1965. Arch. Klin. Exp. Derm. **227**, 913–914 (1966).

81. de Dulanto, F., Sánchez-Muros, J.: Tratamiento quirurgio del cáncer cutaneo-mucoso. In: Jadassohn,W., Schirren, C.G.: XIII. Congressus internat. Dermatologiae, Vol. I. Berlin-Heidelberg-New York: Springer 1968.

82. Dunham, T.: A method of obtaining a skin flap from the scalp and a permanent vascular pedicle for covering defects of the face. Ann. Surg. **17**, 676–679 (1893).

83. Dupuis, C., Rees, T.D.: Historical notes on blepharoplasty. Plast. Reconstr. Surg. **47**, 246–251 (1971).

84. Durau, H.U., Hundeiker, M.: Zur Differentialdiagnostik benigner pigmentierter Hauttumoren. Z. Hautkr. **49**, 301–308 (1974).

85. Eberhartinger, C., Santler, R.: Prognose und Therapie der Lippenkarzinome. Z. Hautkr, **44**, 585–588 (1969).

86. Ebner, H.: Cytostatische Behandlung von Epitheliomen mit einer 5% 5-Fluorouracil-Salbe. Z. Hautkr. **43**, 757–762 (1968).

87. Ebner, H.: Elektronenmikroskopische Un-

tersuchungen über die Wirkung von 5-Fluo-
rouracil auf Basaliome. Z. Hautkr. **46,**
465–472 (1971).

88. Ehlers, G.: Zur Klinik der Basalzellepithe-
liome unter Berücksichtigung statistischer
Untersuchungen. Z. Hautkr. **41,** 226–238
(1966).

89. Edwards, J.M.: Malignant melanoma: Surgical aspects of treatment. Proc. R. Soc.
Med. **65,** 140–144 (1972).

9p. Eidherr, H.: Klinische Erfahrungen mit der
radioaktiven Lymphographie. - Verh.
Dtsch. Dermat. Ges., 29. Tagung, Berlin,
29.9.-2.10. 1971. Arch. Derm. Forsch. **224,**
254–255 (1972).

91. Elliot, R.A.: Rotation flaps of the nose.
Plast. Reconstr. Surg. **44,** 147–149 (1969).

92. Elste, G.: Das Vollhaut-Transplantat in der
korrektiven Dermatologie. Aesthet. Med.
14, 64–73 (1965).

93. Elste, J.: Zur Pathogenese der Chondrodermatitis nodularis chronica helicis. Dermatol. Wochenschr. **130,** 337–384 (1965).

94. Elste, G.: Die operative Behandlung von
Krankheiten und kosmetischen Schäden
der Haut vom Standpunkt des Dermatologen. Aesthet. Med. **15,** 160–166 (1966).

95. Emmet, A.F.F.: The closure of defects by
using adjacent triangular flaps with subcutaneous pedicles. Plast. Reconstr. Surg. **59,**
45–52 (1977).

96. Engeloch, F., Küpter, U.: Kleine Chirurgie
für den praktischen Arzt. Bern-Stuttgart-
Wien: H. Huber 1971.

97. Epker, B.M., Wolford, L.J.: Reduction
cheiloplasty: its role in the correction of
dentofacial deformities. J. Maxillofac. Surg.
5, 134–141 (1977).

98. Epstein, E. (ed.): Skin Surgery, 1st ed. Philadelphia: Lea & Febiger 1956.

99. Epstein, E. (ed.): Skin Surgery, 2nd ed.
Philadelphia: Lea & Febiger 1962.

100. Epstein, E., Pollack, R.S.: General principles of skin surgery. In: Skin Surgery (ed.
E. Epstein), 2nd ed., pp.23–32. Philadelphia: Lea & Febiger 1962.

101. Epstein, E.: An office surgery. In: Skin Surgery (ed. E. Epstein), 2nd ed., pp. 33–34.
Philadelphia: Lea & Febiger 1962.

102. Epstein, E.: Cautery excision. In: Skin Surgery (ed. E. Epstein), 2nd ed., pp. 202–208.
Philadelphia: Lea & Febiger 1962

103. Epstein, N.N.: Electrodessication and curettage. In: Skin Surgery (ed. E. Epstein),

2nd ed., pp. 209–215. Philadelphia: Lea &
Febiger 1962.

104. Epstein, E.: Dermabrasion. In: Skin Surgery (ed. E. Epstein), 2nd ed., pp. 243–267.
Philadelphia: Lea & Febiger 1962.

105. Epstein, E.: The surgical treatment of baldness. In: Skin Surgery (ed. E. Epstein), 2nd
ed., pp. 331–336. Philadelphia: Lea & Febiger 1962.

106. Epstein, E: Cautery surgery. Derm. Dig. **6,**
47–56 (1967).

107. Epstein,E., Epstein, N.N., Bragg, H., Lin-
den, G.: Metastases from squamous cell
carcinomas of the skin. Arch. Dermatol. **97,**
245–251 (1968).

108. Erczy, M., Zoltàn, J.: Spezielle plastische
Chirurgie. Budapest: Medicinae 1958.

109. Esser, J.F.S.: Island flaps. N. Y. Med. J.
106, 264–265 (1917).

110. Esser, J.F.S.: Die Rotation der Wange und
allgemeine Bemerkungen bei chirurgischer
Gesichtsplastik. Leipzig: Vogel 1918.

111. Esser, J.F.S.: Gestielte lokale Nasenplastik
mit zweizipfligen Lappen, Deckung des
sekundären Defekts vom ersten Zipfel durch
den zweiten. Dtsch. Z. Chir. **143.** 385 (1918).

112. Esser, J.F.S.: Biological or Artery Flaps of
the Face. Monaco: Instit. Esser de Chirurg.
Struct. 1934.

113. Estlander, J.A.: Eine Methode, aus der einen Lippe Substanzverluste der anderen zu
ersetzen. Arch. Klin. Chir. **14,** 622–631
(1872).

114. Etschenberg, E.: Anästhesie mit Droperidol
und Fentanyl. Aulendorf: Editio Cantor
1973.

115. Fara, M.: Rhinophym: Erfahrungen bei 81
operierten Patienten. Acta Chir. Plast.
(Praha) **13,** 254–260 (1971).

116. Fischl, R.A.: Vertical abdominoplasty.
Plast. Reconstr. Surg. **51,** 139–143 (1973).

117. Fischer, H.: Die Pathophysiologie und
Funktionsdiagnostik der venösen Durchblu-
tungs störungen. In: Fortsch. Prakt. Derm.
Venerol., Vol. 7 (eds. O.Braun-Falco,
D.Petzoldt), pp. 110–116. Berlin-Heidel-
berg-New York: Springer 1973.

118. Fischer, W.J.: Rhinophyma: its surgical
treatment. Plast. Reconstr. Surg. **45,**
466–470 (1970).

119. Flegel, H.: Möglichkeiten der Kome-
donenentfernung. Aesthet. Med. **15,** 80–82
(1966).

120. Flowers, R.S.: Zigzag blepharoplasty for

upper eyelids. Plast. Reconstr. Surg. **47**, 557–559 (1971).

121. Foussereau, J., Benezra, C.: Les eczémas allergiques professionels. Paris: Masson 1970.

122. Freeman, B.S.: Reconstructive rhinoplasty for rhinophyma. Plast Reconstr. Surg. **46**, 265–270 (1970).

123. Freilinger, G.: Probleme der chirurgischen Behandlung von Tierfellnaevi. Chirurgia plastica **5**, 163–169 (1968).

124. Freilinger, G., Santler, R.: Zur chirurgischen Behandlung maligner Hauttumoren im Nasenbereich. A. Hautkr. **45**, 29–33 (1970).

125. Friederich, H.C.: Aesthetische Geisichtspunkte bei der Entfernung des Hautkarzinoms. Aesthet. Med. **10**, 197–203 (1961).

126. Friederich, H.C.: Korrektive Dermatologie. In: E. Riecke, Lehrbuch der Haut-und Geschlechtskrankheiten. Stuttgart: G. Fischer 1962.

127. Friederich, H.C.: Schwenklappenplastiken. Dermatol. Wochenschr. **150**, 39–53 (1964).

128. Friederich, H.C.: Aktuelle Fragen der Behandlung des Lupus vulgaris. Z. Hautkr. **37**, 163–188 (1964).

129. Friederich, H.C.: Zur Methodik der operativen Entfernung des Unterlippenkarzinoms in Stadium I der Erkrankung nach Eller und Eller. Dermatol. Wochenschr. **150**, 393–407 (1964).

130. Friederich, H.C.: Dauerhaftigkeit, Gefahren und Mißerfolge kosmetischer Eingriffe im Rahmen der korrektiven Dermatologie. Aesthet. Med. **13**, 377–390 (1964).

131. Friederich, H.C.: Zur Frage der konservativen dermatologischen Behandlung von Narben und narbenartigen Zustandsbildern verschiedener Genese. Aesthet. Med. **15**, 260–263 (1966).

132. Friederich, H.C.: Zur Therapie des Rhinophyms. Aesthet. Med. **16**, 169–182 (1967).

133. Friederich, H.C.: Therapieergebnisse beim Unterlippencarcinom (Stadium I nach Eller u. Eller) nach Keilexcision und Schichtnaht. Hautarzt **19**, 168–172 (1968).

134. Friederich, H.C.: Indikationen und Ergebnisse operativplastischer Maßnahmen am dermatologischen Krankengut. Therapiewoche **19**, 1019–1024 (1969).

135. Friederich, H.C.: Indikation und Technik der opperativplastischen Behandlung des Haarverlusts. Hautarzt **21**, 197–202 (1970).

136. Friederich, H.C.: Korrektive Dermatologie. In: Haut- und Geschlechtskrankheiten (eds. Bode, H.B., Korting, G.W.), Vol. 2, pp. 790–801. Stuttgart: G. Fischer 1970.

137. Friederich, H.C.: Die operative Therapie des Haarausfalls. Kosmetologie **1**, 205–206 (1972).

138. Friederich, H.C., Horn,W.: Narben, Keloide und Atrophien des Hautorgans. In: Fortschr. Prakt. Derm. Venerol. (eds. O.Braun-Falco, D.Petzoldt), Vol. 7, pp. 93–101. Berlin-Heidelberg-New York: Springer 1973.

139. Friederich, H.C., Horn, W., Pfitzmann, A.: Atrophien der Haut. Dtsch. Ärztebl. **70**, 3369–3374 (1973).

140. Friederich, H.C., Lehmann, E.: Einzeitige Radikaloperation von Hautcarcinomen des Schädels mit anschließender plastischer Deckung durch Verschiebelappen. Z. Hautkr. **30**, 1–14 (1961).

141. Friederich, H.C., Schneider, H.J.: Ergebnisse der operativen Behandlung der Melanosis circumscripta praeblastomatosa Dubreuilh. Med. Welt (Stuttg.) **17**, 2495–2500 (1966).

142. Friederich, H.C., Schneller, B.: Handrücken-Karzinome aus der Sicht des Dermatologen. Dermatol Wochenschr. **151**, 1175–1188 (1965).

143. Friederich, H.C., Seib, H.: Ergebnisse der Keilexzision aus der Ohrmuschel mit Knorpelentnahme bei der Behandlung der Chondrodermatitis nodularis chronica helicis. Aesthet. Med. **18**, 141–148 (1969).

144. Friederich, H.C., Vakilzadeh, F.: Über die Vermilionektomie. Z. Hautkr **43**, 485-492 (1968).

145. Friederich, H.C., Willmund, G.: Entfermung von Tätowierungen. Dtsch. Ärztebl. **71**, 296–299 (1974).

146. Friederich, H.C.: Defektdeckung von Unterschenkelgeschwüren aus der Sicht des Dermatologen. Z. Hautkr. **49**, 377–381 (1974).

147. Friedrich, H.K., Hundeiker, M.: Klinik und Histologie in der dermatologischen Differential-diagnostik. Arch. Dermatol. Forsch. **250**, 51–64 (1974).

148. Fries, R.: Vorzug der Bernardschen Operation als Universalverfahren zur Rekonstruktion der Unterlippe nach Carcinomresektion. Chir. plastica (Berl.) **1**, 45–52 (1971).

149. Funk, C.Fr.: Zur Decortication des Rhinophyms. Aesthet. Med. 17, 43–44 (1968).
150. Gabka, J.: Ist die chirurgische Hautnaht heute schon entbehrlich? (Klinische und experimentelle Untersuchungen zum Wundnahtverschluβ). Chir. plastica (Berl.) 5, 254–256 (1968).
151. Gartmann, H.: Trauma und malignes Melanom. Hefte Unfallheilkd. 107, 50–52 (1971).
152. Gartmann, H.: Therapie des malignen Melanoms. Dtsch. Med. Wochenschr. 97, 1305–1307 (1972).
153. Gelbke, H.: Die Schnittführung nach Le Mesurier und andere moderne. Gesichtspunkte bei der Operation von Lippenspalten. Bruns' Beitr. Klin. Chir. 188, 406 (1954).
154. Gelbke, H.: Kopf und Gesicht. In: Hellner,H., Nissen,R., Vossschulte, K., Lehrbuch der Chirurgie. Stuttgart: Thieme 1962.
155. Gelbke, H.: Wiederherstellende und plastische Chirurgie, Vols. I-III. Stuttgart: Thieme 1968.
156. Georg, H.: Über die Bedeutung der Flächenspannung bei der freien autologen Vollhaut transplantation. Aesthet. Med. 14, 14–20 (1965).
157. Georgiade, N.G., Mladick, R.A., Thorne, F.L.: The nasolabial tunnel flap. Plast. Reconstr. Surg. 43, 463–466 (1966).
158. Gertler, W.: Praktische Dermatologie. Diagnostische und therapeutische Methoden. Leipzig: VEB G. Thieme 1965.
159. Gibson, D.: Locally malignant and radioresistant tumors of the face. Plast. Reconstr. Surg. 34, 491–500 (1964).
160. Gillies, H.D., Millard, D.R.,Jr.: Principles and Art of Plastic Surgery. Boston: Little, Brown & Co. 1957.
161. Glass, R.L.: Skin cancer. Principles of management. Missouri Med. 62, 194–295 (1965).
162. Glass, R.L., Spratt, J.S., Perez-Mesa, C.: The fate of inadequately excised epidermoid carcinoma of the skin. Surg. Gynecol. Obstet. 122, 245–248 (1966).
163. Go, M.J., Delemarre, J.F.M., Hundeiker, M.: Zur Frage der Metastasierung des Basalzell-epithelioms („Basalzellcarcinoms"). Hautarzt 24, 449–451 (1973).
164. Göltner, E.: Ungewöhnlicher Verlauf eines Keratoakanthoms nach Fräsbehandlung. Aesthet. Med. 9, 269–272 (1960).
165. Götz, H.: Indikationen zur Verödungsbehandlung der Varizen. In: Fortschr. Prakt.

Derm. Venerol., Vol. 7 (eds. O.Braun-Falco, D. Petzoldt), pp. 128–134. Berlin-Heidelberg-New York: Springer 1973.
166. Gohrbandt, E., Gabka, J., Berndorfer, A.: Handbuch der plastischen Chirurgie. Berlin: W. de Gruvter 1968.
167. Goldschmidt, H.: Kurettage und Elektrodesikkation bei Basaliom, spinozellularem Karzinom und Keratoakanthom. Fortschr. Prakt. Derm. Venerol. Vol. 8 (ed. O. Braun-Falco, S. Marghescu), pp. 41–48. Berlin-Heidelberg-New York: Springer 1976.
168. Goldsmith, H.S., Shan, J.P., Kim, D.H.: Prognostic significance of lymph node dissection in the treatment of malignant melanoma. Cancer (Philad.) 26, 606–609 (1970).
169. Gorney, M., Falces, E., Jones, H., Manis, J.R.: One-stage reconstruction of substantial lower eye lid margin defects. Plast. Reconstr. Surg. 44, 592–596 (1969).
170. Gottron, H.A., Nikolowski, W.: Karzinom der Haut. In: Gottron, H.A., Schönfeld, W., Dermatologie und Venerologie, Vol. IV. Stuttgart: Thieme 1960.
171. Grabb, W.C. Myers, W.B. (eds.): Skin Flaps. Boston: Little, Brown & Co 1975.
172. Grazer, F.M.: Abdominoplasty. Plast. Reconstr. Surg. 51, 617–623 (1973).
173. Gregl, A.: Die Lymphographie in ihrer diagnostischen und therapeutischen Bedeutung für das maligne Melanom. Verh. Dtsch. Dermat. Ges., 29. Tagung, Berlin, 29.9–2.10. 1971. Arch. Dermatol. Forsch. 244, 241–245 (1972).
174. Greither, A.: Indikationen zur operativen Behandlung von Varizen. In: Fortschr. prakt. Derm. Venerol. (eds. O. Braun-Falco, D. Petzoldt), Vol. 7, pp. 122–127. Berlin-Heidelberg-New York: Springer 1973.
175. Greither, A., Tritsch, H.: Die Geschwülste der Haut. Ihr klinisches und feingewebliches Bild, ihre Erkennung und Behandlung. Stuttgart: G.Thieme 1957.
176. Griffith, B.H., McKinney, P.: An appraisal of the treatment of basal cell carcinoma of the skin. Plast. Reconstr. Surg. 51, 565–574 (1973).
177. Grimm, G.: Die Invagination der oberen Ohrmuschel—eine seltene Miβbildung und ihre plastische Korrektur. Aesthet. Med. 10, 59–61 (1961).
178. Grützmacher, K.Th.: Beitrag zur Frage des Röntgenkarzinoms. Strahlentherapie 72, 330–336 (1943).

179. Gründer, K., Leyh, F.: Lokale Behandlung von Hauttumoren mit 5%iger Fluorouracilsalbe. Hautarzt 23, 217–221 (1972).
180. Gründer, B., Hundeiker, M.: Keratoakanthom und Karzinom. Dermatol. Monatschr. 159, 122–133 (1973).
181. Günther, H.: Lippenschleimhautersatz im Rahmen der Rekonstruktion der Unterlippe. Zentralbl. Dtsch. Zahn- u. Kieferheilkd. 47, 321–332 (1966).
182. Günther, H., Spiessl, B.: Rekonstruktionen der Unterlippe nach Carcinomentfernung und gleichzeitiger Austräumung regionärer Lymphknoten. Chir. plastica (Berl.) 3, 230–240 (1967).
183. Haas, E.: Chirurgische Behandlung von Lippentumoren. Z. Laryng. Rhinol. 44, 276–291 (1965).
184. Haasters, J.: Operative Eingriffe in der Dermatologie. Inaug.-Diss. Freiburg i. Br. 1969.
185. Hagedorn, M., Petres, F.: Nahplastik am Rücken (Indikation und Technik). Acta Chir. Maxillo-facialis Vol.2, pp. 137–141. F.A. Barth: Leipfig 1977.
186. Haid-Fischer, F., Haid, H.: Venenerkrankungen. Phlebologie für Klinik und Praxis, 3rd ed. Vol. I/II. Stuttgart: Thieme 1973.
187. Happle, R.: Surgical treatment of erythroplasia of Queyrat. Plast. Reconstr. Surg. 59, 642–645 (1977).
188. Harris, M.N., Cumport, S.L. Berman, I.R., Bernard, R.W.: Ilioinguinal lymph node dissection for melanoma. Surg. Gynecol. Obstet. 136, 33–39 (1973).
188a. Hartmann, M., Petres, J.: Hautartz 29, 82–85 (1978).
189. Hegmann, G.: Allgemeine Operationslehre. In: Allgemeine und spezielle chirurgische Operationslehre, begr. v. M. Kirschner, 2nd ed. (eds. N.Guleke, R. Zenker), Vol. I, Part 1. Berlin-Göttingen-Heidelberg: Springer 1958.
190. Heite, H.-J.: Bericht über das Symposion „Malignes Melanom", veranstaltet von der Deutschen Forschungsgemeinschaft am 4./5.6.1962 in Freiburg i. Br. Hautarzt 14, 554–561 (1963).
191. Helm, F.: The treatment of carcinoma of the skin. Manitoba Med. Rev. 45, 349–350 (1965).
192. Helm, F., Milgrom, H., Phelan, J.T., Klein, E.: Zur chemochirurgischen Behandlung der Hautkarzinome. Chemochirurgische Methode (nach Mohs) einer mikroskopisch kontrollierten Behandlung von Hautkreb-

sen. Dermatol Wochenschr. 150, 451—458 (1964).
193. Hernández-Richter, J., Jacobi, W.: Kombination von Schwenklappenplastik und Spalthaut-transplantation bei der Deckung größerer Weichteildefekte am Schädel. Chir. Praxis 7, 253 (1963).
194. Herrmann, A.: Gefahren bei Operationen am Hals, Ohr und Gesicht und die Korrektur fehlerhafter Eingriffe. Berlin-Heidelberg-New York: Springer 1968.
195. Herrmann, J.B.: Moderne chirurgische Nahtmaterialien: Ihre Eigenschaften und Anwendung. In: International Symposium: Sutures in wound repair. London, July 10–11, 1972. Deutsche Fassung: Redaktion Ethicon op forum.
196. Hertig, P.: Une nouvelle technique de reconstruction plastique de la lèvre inférieure. Pract. oto-rhino-laryng. (Basel) 27, 157–166 (1965).
197. Hoffmeister, H.E.: Kie chirurgische Behandlung der Beinvarizen. Z. Hautkr 49, 389–391 (1974).
198. Holland, G., Bellmann, O.: Zur Klinik und Therapie der Basaliome und Spinaliome. Ophthalmologica (Basel) 150, 138–152 (1965).
199. Hollmann, K.: Zur chirurgischen Behandlung maligner Geschwülste der Unterlippe. Öst. Z. 62, 202–204 (1965).
200. Hollwich, F., Jünemann, G.: Defektdekung nach Entfernung von Lidtumoren. Chir. plastica (Berl.) 3, 200–208 (1967).
201. Holström, H.: Surgical treatment of malignant melanomas (in Swedish). Nord. Med. 85, 507 (1971).
202. Honeycutt, W.M., Janssen, G.T.: Treatment of squamous cell carcinoma of the skin. Arch. Dermatol. 108, 670–672 (1973).
203. Horn, W.: Ergebnisse des niedertourigen Hautschliffes bei seborrhoischen Warzen. Z. Hautkr. 48, 971–974 (1973).
204. Hueston, J.T.: Integumentectomy for malignant melanoma of the limbs. Aust. N.Z.J. Surg. 40, 114–118 (1970).
205. Huffstadt, A.J.C.: Vergrößerung der Fläche freier Hauttransplantate. Z. Kinderchir. 11, Suppl., 320–324 (1972).
206. Huffstadt, A.J.C.: Zit. nach J. Hernández-Richter, Chir. plastica (Berl.) 3, 163–167 (1967).
207. Hundeiker, M., Mulert, L.,v.: Vermeidbare Risiken bei der Hodenbiopsie. Hautarzt 17, 546–547 (1966).

208. Hundeiker, M.: Warum ist die „hohe Unterbindung" nach Palomo und nicht eine Varicocelenoperation schlechthin Methode der Wahl zur Behandlung durch Varicocelen bedingter Fertilitätsstörungen? Hautarzt **21**, 37–38 (1970).

209. Hundeiker, M., Brehm, K.: Naevus flammeus und Hämangiom. Fortschr. Med. **91**, 855–856 (1973).

210. Hundeiker, M., Gründer, B., Junge, K.-G.: Lokalisation und Alterverteilung der Keratomata solaria. Arch. Dermatol. Forsch. **247**, 373–378 (1973).

211. Illig, L.: Moderne, kombinierte Melanom-Therapie. Akt. Dermatol. **2**, 1–25 (1976).

212. Imre, J.: Lidplastik und plastische Operation anderer Weichteile des Gesichtes. Budapest: Studium-Verlag 1928.

213. Imre, J.: Operationen an den Lidern. In: Ophthalmologische Operationslehre (ed. R. Thiel). Leipzig: Thieme 1942.

214. Ingram, R.C., Krantz, S., Mandeloff, J., Leslie, H.: Some observations on carcinoma of the lip. Oral Surg. **19**, 684–690 (1965).

215. Ivanissevich, O.: Left varicocele due to reflux; experience with 4470 operative cases in forty-two years. J. Int. Coll. Surg. **34**, 742–755 (1960).

216. Johnson, J.B., Hadley, R.C.: The aging face. In: Plastic and reconstructive surgery (ed. J.M. Converse), Vol. 3: The head and neck. Philadelphia: W.B. Saunders 1964.

217. Jones, H.W., Kahn, R.A.: Surgical treatment of elephantiasis of the male genitalia. Plast. Reconstr. Surg. **46**, 8–12 (1970).

218. Jones, R.F., Dickinson, W.E.: Total integumentectomy of the leg for multiple „intransit" metastases of melanoma. Am. J. Surg. **123**, 588–590 (1973).

219. Joseph, J.: Nasenplastik und sonstige Gesichts plastik. Leipzig: C. Kabitzsch 1932.

220. Jost, G., Legent, F., Méresse, B.: Atlas der aesthetischen plastischen Chirurgie. Stuttgart-New York: F.K. Schattaner 1977.

221. Junge, K.G., Hundeiker, M.: Histologische Untersuchungen an „Cornua cutanea". Dermatol Monatsschr. **159**, 619–630 (1973).

222. Kärcher, K.H.: Zur Problematik der Therapie kindlicher Angiome. Fortschr. Med. **86**, 1028–1030 (1968).

223. Kalkoff, K.W.: Über die Sonderstellung des Lupuskarzinoms unter Berücksichtigung der Konsequenzen für Therapie and Pro-

phylaxe. Strahlentherapie **86**, 468–476 (1952).

224. Kalkoff, K.W.: Hauterscheinungen der Sarkoidose. Internist (Berl.) **10**, 376–380 (1969).

225. Kalkoff, K.W.: Entartungsrisiko des Naevuszellnaevus. Dtsch. Med. Wochenschr. **96**, 399–400 (1971).

226. Kalkoff, K.W.: Naevus flammeus und Hämangiom. Dtsch. Med. Wochenschr. **97**, 353–354 (1972).

227. Kalkoff, K.W.: Zur Klassifizierung und Differentialdiagnose des malignen Melanoms. 2.: Differentialdiagnose des malignen Melanoms. Fortschr. Med. **91**, 1209–1213 (1973).

228. Kalkoff, K.W., Kühnl-Petzoldt, Ch.: Zur Abgrenzung der Melanosis circumscripta praeblastomatosa Dubreuilh vom superficial spreading melanoma und zur Klassifizierung der Melanome. Hautarzt **24**, 463–469 (1973).

229. Kalkoff, K.W., Kühnl-Petzoldt, Ch.: Melanom: Klassifikation nach Clark und prognostische Gesichtspunkte. Diagnostik **7**, 227–231 (1974).

230. Kalkoff, P., Baumeister, L., Gehring, D.: Endolymphatische Radionuklidtherapie bei malignen Melanomen der unteren Extremitäten. Arch. Dermatol. Forsch. **244**, 250–254 (1972).

231. Kalkoff, K.W.: Zur Differentialdiagnose Angiektasia eruptiva thrombotica (Syn. Angiokeratoma, thrombosed Angioma, l'angiome noir) und malignes Melanom. Dermatol Monatschr. **160**, 621–630 (1974).

232. Karge, H.J.: Rhinophym. Dermatochirurgische Möglichkeiten Zur Behandlung. In: Dermatochirurgie in Klinik und Praxis (eds. B. Konz, G. Burg), pp. 195–201. Berlin-Heidelberg-New York: Springer 1977.

233. Kastenbauer, E., Jahnke, O.: Zur Problematik maligner Lippentumoren und deren operative Behandlung. In: Plastische Chirurgie des Kopf-und Halsbereichs und der weiblichen Brust (ed. H. Bohmert). Stuttgart: G. Thieme 1975.

234. Kazanjian, V.H., Converse, J.M.: The surgical treatment of facial injuries, 2nd ed. Baltimore: Williams & Wilkins 1959.

235. Kaya Cilingiroglu, H.: Die Behandlung des Karzinoms der Unterlippe nach der Methode von S. Dirvana Zentralbl. Chir. **91**, 857–861 (1966).

236. Keining, E., Braun-Falco, O.: Dermatolo-

gie und Venerologie, 2nd ed. München: J.F. Lehmann 1969.

237. Kelly, H.A.: Excision of the fat of the abdominal wall—lipectomy. Surg. Gynecol. Obstet. **10**, 229–321 (1910).

238. Kernahan, D.A.: In: W.C. Grabb, J.W. Smith, Plastic Surgery. London: J. & A. Churchill 1968.

239. Kirschner, M.: Allgemeine und spezielle chirurgische Operationslehre, 2nd ed. Vol. IV. Berlin-Göttingen-Heidelberg: Springer 1956.

240. Kleine-Natrop, H.-E.: Die operative Therapie des Dermatologen. Beiträge zur modernen Therapie. Vorträge und Diskussionsbemerkungen der 7. Weimarer Therapietagung 1961 sowie Originalarbeiten und Übersichtsreferate (ed. G.P. Hesse) Jena: G. Fischer 1962.

241. Kligman, A.M., Christophers, E.: Preparation of isolated sheets of human stratum corneum. Arch. Dermatol. (Chic.) **88**, 702–705 (1963).

242. Knox, J.M., Freeman, R.G.: Treatment of skin cancer. Geriatrics **18**, 654–658 (1963).

243. Knox, J.M., Freemann, R.G., Duncan, W.C., Heaton, C.L.: Treatment of skin cancer. Sth. Med. J. (Bgham, Ala.) **60**, 241–246 (1967).

244. Körner, W.: Die operative Behandlung von Krankheiten und kosmetischen Schäden der Haut vom Standpunkt des Chirurgen. Aesthet. Med. **15**, 167–173 (1966).

245. Krause, F.: Über die Transplantation großer ungestielter Hautlappen. Arch. Klin. Chir. **46**, 177–182 (1893).

246. Krauspe, C., Stelzner, F.: Die Pyodermitis fistulans sinifica. Über die klinischen und histologisch-pathologischen Veränderungen bei einer fistelnden Dermatitis nebst Bemerkungen über die Beziehungen zur sog. Hidradenitis suppurativa bzw. zur Akne conglobata. Chirurg **33**, 534–538 (1962).

247. Krieger, K.: Die subcutane Varizenligatur. Z. Hautkr. **49**, 383–388 (1974).

248. Kromayer, E.: Rotationsinstrumente. Ein neues technisches Verfahren in der dermatologischen Kleinchirurgie. Dermatol. Z. **12**, 26–36 (1905).

249. Kromayer, E.: Die Heilung der Akne durch ein neues narbenloses Operationsverfahren: das Stanzen. Münch. Med. Wochenschr. **52**, 942–944 (1905).

250. Kromayer, E.: Die Behandlung der kosmetischen Hautleiden unter besonderer Berücksichtigung der physikalischen Heilmethoden und der narbenlosen Operationsweisen. Leipzig: G. Thieme 1923.

251. Krüger, E.: Zur Deckung durchgehender Lippen- und Wangendefekte. Chir. Plastica, (Berl.) **1**, 34–44 (1971).

252. Kühl, M.: Chirurgisch-kosmetische Indikationen in Jugend und Alter. Aesthet. Med. **17**, 251–254 (1968).

253. Kurth, M.E.: Lip shave or vermilionectomy: indications and technique. Br. J. Plast. Surg. **10**, 156–162 (1958).

254. Kúta, A.: Über die chirurgische Behandlung der Basaliome unter besonderer Berücksichtigung des kosmetischen Erfolges. Cosmetologica **19**, 123–130 (1970).

255. Kvorning, S.A.: Late results of radiotherapy in cancer of the skin. Acta Derm.-Venereol (Stockh.) **39**, 477–480 (1959).

256. Laake, Ch.: Hochtouriges Schleifen der Hait und Turbinenantrieb. Aesthet. Med **13**, 182–186 (1964).

257. Laake, Ch.: Aesthetische Gesichtspunkte beider operativen Behandlung von Epitheliomen im Gesichts-Kopf-Bereich im Rahmen der Dermatologie. Aesthet. Med. **13**, 261–266 (1964).

258. Landes, E.: Zur operativen Behandlung der Hyperhidrosis axillaris. In: Dermatochirurgie in Klinik und Praxis (eds. B. Konz, G. Burg) pp. 178–182. Berlin-Heidelberg-New York: Springer 1977.

259. Langenbeck, B.V.: Neues Verfahren zur Cheiloplastic durch Ablösung und Verziehung des Lippensaumes. Deutsche Klinik **7**, 1–3 (1855).

260. Langenbeck, B.V., Zit nach, Joseph J.: Nasenplastik und sonstige Gesichtsplastik. Leipzig: C. Kabitzsch 1932.

261. Laugier, P., Orusco, M., Wagenknecht, L., Jaccard, M.A.: Polychimiothérapie du mélanomemétastatique. Soc. Suisse Derm. Véner., 53e Réunion ann., Bâle 1971. Dermatologica (Basel) **145**, 72–79 (1972).

262. Le Coulant, P., Maleville, J., Cardinand, J.P.: La radiothérapie superficielle sans filtre en une seánce dans le traitement des cancers cutanés (methode de W. Dubreuilh). Dermatologia (Napoli) **12**, 65–76 (1961).

263. Lehmann, A., Jr., Garret, W.S., Jr., Musgrav, Ross H.: Earlobe composite grafts for the correction of nasal defects. Plast. Reconstr. Surg. **47**, 12–16 (1971).

264. Lentrodt, J.: Neubildungen in Kieferbereich: Diagnostische Probleme des Haus-
und Zahnarztes. Diagnostik 6, 745–749
(1973).
265. Lentrodt, F.: Principles of the surgical therapy of eyelid tumours. J. Maxillofac. Surg.
5, 93–107 (1977).
266. Lewis, K.G., Landa, S.: Radiation burns.
J. Int. Coll. Surg. 37, 237–259 (1962).
267. Limberg, A.A.: Design of local flaps. In: T.
Gibson, Modern Trends in Plastic Surgery.
Washington: Butterworth 1966.
268. Limberger, S., Dietz, H., Boepple, D.: Beitrag zur Behandlung von Hautkarzinom-Re-
zidiven nach Röntgenvorbestrahlung. Dermatol Wochenschr. 152, 201–208 (1966).
269. Lincoln, C.S., Nordstrom, R.C.: Scalpel
scissors surgery. In: Skin Surgery (ed. E.
Epstein), 2nd ed., pp. 45–91. Philadelphia:
Lea & Febiger 1962.
270. Lindemann, A., Lange, G., Frenzel, H.:
Die Chirurgie des Gesichts, der Mundhöhle
und der Luftwege. Berlin-Vienna: Urban
& Schwarzenberg 1941.
271. Lister, G.D., Gibson, T.: Closure of rhom-
boid skin defects: the flaps of Limberg and
Dufourmentel. Brit. J. Plast. Surg. 47, 33–36
(1971).
272. Loeb, R.: Esthetic blepharoplasty based on
the degree of wrinkling. Plast Reconstr.
Surg. 47, 33–36 (1971).
273. Loney II, W.R.R.: Chemosurgical treatment of skin cancer. J. Okla. Med. Ass. 60,
165–168 (1967).
274. Longenecker, C.G., Ryan, R.F.: Cancer of
the lip in a large charity hospital Sth. Med.
J. (Bgham, Ala.) 58, 1459–1460 (1965).
275. Lopez-Mas, J., Oritz-Monasterio, F., de
Gonzalez, M.V., Olmedo, A.: Skin graft
pigmentation. A new approach to prevention. Plast. Reconstr. Surg. 49, 18–21 (1972).
276. Lueders, H.W.: Regional nasal flaps. In:
Conley, J., Dickinson, J.T.: Plastic and Reconstructive Surgery of the Face and Neck,
Vol. II. Stuttgart: Thieme 1972.
277. Lueders, H.W., Shapiro, R.L.: Rotation
finger flaps in reconstruction of burned
hands. Plast. Reconstr. Surg. 47, 176–178
(1971).
278. Lynch, G.A.: Cancer of the lip. Ulster Med.
J. 36, 44–50 (1967).
279. McBride, C.M.: Perfusion treatment for
malignant melanoma of the extremity. Arch.
Chir. Neerl. 22, 91–95 (1970).
280. Macher, E.: Einleitung zum Thema II: Der-
zeitiger Stand der Immunologie des malignen Melanoms. 105. Tagung der Vereini-

gung der Südwestdeutschen Dermatologen
gemeinsam mit der Vereinigung Rheinisch-
Westfälischer Dermatologen, Freiburg i.
Br. 20.–21.4. 1974.
281. McCallum, D.I., Kinmont, P.D.C.: Basal
cell carcinoma. An analysis of cases seen at
a combined clinic. Br. J. Dermatol 78,
141–146 (1966).
282. McGregor, J.A.: Fundamental Techniques
of Plastic Surgery and Their Surgical Application. Edinburgh and London: E. & S.
Livingstone 1960
283. McInnes, G.F., Freeman, J.M., Engler,
H.S.: Control of basal cell carcinoma. 10
year review. Am. J. Surg. 31, 828–830
(1965).
284. McKee, D.M.: Treatment of basal cell carcinoma. South Med. J. 209–215 (1964).
285. Madsen, A.: The histogenesis of superficial
basal cell epitheliomas. Arch. Dermatol. 72,
29–30 (1955).
286. May, H.: Reconstructive and reparative
surgery. Phildelphia: F.A. Davis 1949.
287. Melching, H.J.: Radiobiologie. In: Knierer,
W., Praktische Strahlentherapie. Stuttgart:
Medica Verlag 1957.
288. Menning, H.: Über Defektdeckung strah-
lengeschädigter Haut im Gesichts- und
Halsbereich. Hautarzt 18, 264–268 (1967).
289. Meyer, R.: Dauerhaftigkeit, Gefahren und
Mißerfolge kosmetischer Eingriffe im Gesichtsbereich. Aesthet. Med. 13, 273–284
(1964).
290. Meyer, R.: Diskussionsbemerkung zu H.C.
Friederich: Dauerhaftigkeit, Gefahren und
Mißerfolge kosmetischer Eingriffe im Rahmen der kosmetischen Dermatologie. Aesthet. Med. 13, 377–394 (1964).
291. Meyer, R.: Die plastischen Operationsmethoden bei der Formkorrektur des alternden Antlitzes. Aesthet. Med. 13, 19–28
(1967).
292. Meyer, R.: Sekundärplastik nach Verbrennungsschäden der Nase und der Ohren.
Chir. Plastica (Berl.) 1, 135–142 (1966).
293. Meyer, R.: Plastiche Chirurgie bei Anoma-
lien, Defekten und Narben. Aesthet. Med.
17, 229–232 (1968).
294. Meyer-Rohn, J.: Kokkenerkrankungen. In:
Dermatologie und Venerologie (eds. Gottron, H.A., Schönfeld, W.), Vol. II, Part 2.
Stuttgart: Thieme 1958.
295. Meyer-Rohn, J., Fritzemeier, C.U.: Zur
Entfernung von Tätowierungen. Hautarzt
25, 9–12 (1974).
296. Meszaros, C., Nagy, E., Szodoray, L.: Die
Behandlung von Basaliomen mit Colcemid

und Colchicin. Z. Hautkr. **41**, 64–71 (1966).

297. Mihm, M.C.: Kriterien der Klassifikation. 105. Tagung der Vereinigung der Südwestdeutschen Dermatologen gemeinsam mit der Vereinigung Rheinisch- Westfälischer Dermatologen, Freiburg i. Br. 20.–21.4. 1974.

298. Miller, R.F.: „Dermabrasion" mit rotierenden Drahtbürsten in den Vereinigten Staaten. Behandlung eines Falles von Lichen sclerosus et atrophicus. Med. Kosmetik **6**, 217–220 (1957).

299. Milton, S.H.: Experimental studies on island flaps. Plast. Reconstr. Surg. **48**, 574–578 (1971).

300. Mir y Mir, L.: The six-flap Z-plasty. Plast. Reconstr. Surg. **52**, 625–628 (1973).

301. Mitchell, J.C., Hardie, M.: Treatment of basal cell carcinoma by curettage and electrosurgery. Can. Med. Ass. J. **93**, 349–352 (1965).

302. Mohs, F.E.: Chemosurgery in cancer gangrene and infection. Springfield, Ill.: Ch.C Thomas 1956.

303. Mohs, F.E.: The chemosurgical method for the mikroscopically controlled excision of cutaneous cancer. In: Skin Surgery (ed. E. Epstein) 2nd ed., pp. 223–242. Philadelphia: Lea & Febiger 1962.

304. Moldenhauer, E.: Operative Behandlung der Follikulitis nuchae sclerotisans. Aesthet. Med. **13**, 188–192 (1964).

305. Moldenhauer, E.: Zur Technik und Indikation der Z-Plastik. Aesthet. Med. **15**, 362–365 (1966).

306. Moncorps, C.: Subkutane Schlitzung der Talgdrüsen, eine Behandlungsmethode der Akne vulgaris. Münch. Med. Wochenschr. **76**, 997–998 (1929).

307. Moncorps, C.: Über die Beseitigung ausgedehnter Fremdkörpereinsprengungen in der Haut mittels kombinierten Fräs-Ätzverfahrens. Münch. Med. Wochenschr. **89**, 587–588 (1942).

308. Monks, G.H.: restoration of the lower eyelids by a new method. Boston. Med. Surg. J. **139**, 385–387 (1898).

309. Moore, J.R.: Treatment of cicatrizing basal cell carcinomas. Plast. Reconstr. Surg. **47**, 371–374 (1971).

310. Moragas, J.M. de, Gimenez-Camarasa, J.M.: 5-Flourouracil ointment in tumors of the skin. Dermatologica (Basel) **140**, Suppl. 1, 65–74 (1970).

311. Morfit, H.M., Cohen, B.I., Ratzer, E.R.: End results in melanoma. Cancer (Philad.) **22**, 945–948 (1968).

312. Morgan, B.L., Samiian, M.R.: Advantages of the bilobed flap closure of small defects of the face. Plast. Reconstr. Surg. **52**, 35–37 (1973).

313. Moser, M.H., DiPirro, E., McCoy, F.J.: Sudden blindness following blepharoplasty. Report of seven cases. Plast. Reconstr. Surg. **51**, 364–370 (1973).

314. Mouly, R.: Correction of hypertrophy of the upper lip. Plast. Reconstr. Surg. **46**, 262–264 (1970).

315. Müller, R.F.G.: Über die Nasenplastik der alten indischen Ärzte. Chir. Plastica (Berl.) **2**, 12–15 (1966).

316. Mullins, J.F.: Surgical treatment of chronic hidradenitis suppurativa. In: Skin Surgery (ed. E. Epstein), 2nd ed., pp. 326–330. Philadelphia: Lea & Febiger 1962.

317. Mustardé, J.C.: Repair and Reconstruction in the Orbital Region. Edinburgh: E. & S. Livingstone 1966.

318. Mustardé, J.C.: Surgical treatment of malignant tumors of the upper lip. Chir. Plastica (Berl.) **1**, 25–33 (1971).

319. Nagel, F.: Die rekonstruktive und korrektive Chirurgie der äußeren Nase. Dtsch. Ärztebl. **70**, 3118–3123 (1973).

320. Naumann, H.H.: Funktionelle Geisichtspunkte bei Nasenplastiken. Chir. Plastica (Berl.) **5**, 204–211 (1968).

321. Nelson, L.M.: Podophyllin-salicylic acid solution in treatment of basal cell carcinomas. Arch. Dermatol. **93**, 457–459 (1966).

322. Neumann, E.: Behandlung von Onychomykosen durch Nagelablation unter Anwendung von Hyaluronidase. Dermatol. Wochenschr. **136**, 746–748 (1957).

323. Nicolau, S.G., Balus, L.: Chronic actinic cheilitis and cancer of the lower lip. Br. J. Dermatol **76**, 278–289 (1964).

324. Nigst, H.: Chirurgie in der täglichen Praxis. Stuttgart: Hippokrates 1965.

325. Nödl, F.: Die Bedeutung des Mesenchyms für die Wuchsform und die Strahlungsempfindlichkeit des Basalioms. I.-III. Mitteilung. Strahlentherapie **88**, 206–216, 217–227, 228–238 (1952).

326. Nödl, F.: Das echte Randrezidiv und das sukzessive diskontinuierliche Randwachstum des Basalioms nach Röntgeneinwirkung. Strahlentherapie **90**, 265–279 (1953).

327. Nödl, F.: Das sogenannte übergangsepitheliom. I.-IV. Mitteilung. Arch. Dermatol. Syph. (Berl.) **197**, 256-270 (1954).

328. Nödl, F.: Das sogenannte Granuloma teleangiektaticum. Z. Hautkr. **19**, 163–167 (1955).

329. Nödl, F.: Neues auf dem Gebiet der dermatologischen Onkologie. Dtsch. Med. J. **23**, 139–141 (1972).

330. Nolte, H.: Die Technik der Lokalanaesthesie. Berlin-Heidelberg-New York: Springer 1966.

331. Noster, U., Schlosser, G.A., Jänner, M.: Pyodermia fistulans sinifica. Z. Hautkr, **49**, 253–260 (1974).

332. O'Hollovan, M.J.: Skin cancer in Ireland. J. Irish Med. Ass. **60**, 209–213 (1967).

333. Olsen, G.: Some views on the treatment of melanomas of the skin. Arch. Chir. Neerl. **22**, 79–90 (1970).

334. Orentreich, N.: Autografts in alopecias and other selected dermatological conditions. Ann. N.Y. Acad. Sci. **83**, 436 (1959).

335. Ott, F.: Erfahrungen mit der 5-FU-Lokalbehandlung von Präkanzerosen und Karzinomen der Haut.—Schweiz. Ges. Dermatol. Vener., 52. Jahrestagung, Zürich 1970. Dermatologica (Basel) **142**, 276–279 (1971).

336. Pack, G.T., Davis, J.: Radiation cancer of the skin. Radiology **84**, 436–442 (1965).

337. Padgett, E.C.: Surgical Diseases of the Mouth and Jaws. Philadelphia and London: W.B. Saunders 1942.

338. Paletta, F.X.: Lower eyelid reconstruction. Plast. Reconstr. Surg. **51**, 653–657(1973).

339. Palomo, A.: Radical cure of varicocele by a new technique: preliminary report. J. Urol. (Baltimore) **61**, 604–607 (1949).

340. Paul, E.: Eine neue Methode zur Beuteilung der Vitalität von Melanommetastasen nach ,, heißer Lymphographie'' (Ausstellung). 105. Tagung der Vereinigung der Südwestdeutschen Dermatologen gemeinsam mit der Vereinigung Rheinisch- Westfälischer Dermatologen, Freiburg i.Br. 20.–21.4. 1974.

341. Paul, E., Illig, L.: Fluoreszenzmikroskopische Darstellung pigmentbildender Hauttumoren nach Falck-Hillarp im Vergleich zu ihrem gewöhnlichen lichtmikroskopischen Bild. Arch. Dermatol Forsch. **249**, 51–64 (1974).

342. Paul. E., Illig. L.: Fluoreszenzhistochemische Untersuchungen zur Melanomklassifizierung. 9. Symposion der Arbeitsgemeinschaft ,,Malignes Melanom'' der Deutschen Forschungsgemeinschaft, Freiburg 19.4. 1974.

343. Perras, C.: Le traitement de l'épithélioma basocellulaire de la face. Union Med. Can. **94**, 777–780 (1965).

344. Petres, J.: Krankendemonstrationen 39–46. Verh. Dtsch. Dermat. Ges., 27. Tagung, Freiburg 27.9.–3.10. 1965. Arch. Klin. Exp. Dermatol. **227**, 896–897 (1966).

345. Petres, J.: Operative Therapie von Hauttumoren, Vortrag am Fortbildungsseminar der Bezirksärztekammer Südbaden und der Universitäts-Hautklinik, Freiburg i.Br. 28.10. 1967.

346. Petres, J.: Operative Behandlung von Lidtumoren. Z. Hautkr **44**, 29–36 (1969).

347. Petres, J.: Defektdeckung nach operativer Entfernung von karzinomatösen und präblastomatösen Prozessen im Nasenbereich. Aesthet. Med. **18**, 3–8 (1969).

348. Petres, J.: Hautverschiebungen in der Behandlung von Hauttumoren. Vortrag vor der Tagung der Mittelrheinischen Chirurgen in Ludwigshafen/Rhein am 9.10. 1970. Bruns, Beitr. Klin. Chir. **218**, 667 (1971).

349. Petres, J.: Erfahrungen mit plastisch-operativen Maßnahmen in der Behandlung von Hauttumoren. Verh. Dtsch. Dermat. Ges., 29. Tagung, Berlin 29.9.–2.10. 1971. Arch. Dermatol Forsch. **244**, 156–159 (1972).

350. Petres, J.: Zur plastischen Defektdeckung nach Exzision von Hauttumoren. Hautarzt **23**, 271–274 (1972).

351. Petres, J., Haasters, J.: Unterlippenkarzinome—Ein Beitrag zur Therapie. Fortschr. Med. **86**, 785–798 (1968).

352. Petres, J., Haasters, J.: Zur Defektdeckung nach Tumorentfernung im Wangenbereich. Aesthet. Med. **18**, 49–54 (1969).

353. Petres, J., Haasters, J.: Zur operativen Behandlung fortgeschrittener Carcinome und Präcancerosen der Unterlippe. Hautarzt **20**, 219–222 (1969).

354. Petres, J., Haasters, J.: Defektdeckung nach operativer Entfernung von karzinomatösen und praeblastomatösen Prozessen im Nasenbereich. Aesthet. Med. **18**, 3–8 (1969).

355. Petres, J., Haasters, J.: Zur operativen Therapie von Röntgenspätschäden der Haut. Aesthet. Med. **18**, 109–114 (1969).

356. Petres, J., Hagedorn, M.: Behandlung und Prophylaxe von Rezidiven der Papillomatosis cutis carcinoides Gottron mit Bleomycin. Z. Hautkr. **49**, 335–339 (1974).

357. Petres, J., Hagedorn, M.: Zur operativen Therapie ausgedehnter Hauttumoren des Stamms. Hautarzt **25**, 566–569 (1974).

358. Petres, J., Hundeiker, M.: Ein Beitrag zur Therapie beim chronischen Lymphoedem. Z. Hautkr. **43**, 29–31 (1968).

359. Petres, J., Vibrans, U.: Zur operativen Therapie der axillären Hidradenitis suppurativa. Hautarzt **23**, 160–163 (1972).

360. Petres, J.: Zur plastisch-operativen Wundversorgung nach Excision von Lippentumoren. Acta Chir. Maxillofacialis Vol. 1, pp. 18–21. Leipzig: J. A. Barth 1975.

361. Petres, J., Hagedorn, M.: Die Wangenrotation nach Imre. Akt. Dermatol. **2**, 203–207 (1976).

362. Petres, J.: Dermabrasion. In: Dermatochirurgie in Klinik und Praxis, ed. by B. Konz and G. Burg, pp. 211–213. Berlin-Heidelberg-New York: Springer 1977.

363. Petres, J., Hartmann, M., Hagedorn, M.: Unterlippen-Karzinome und deren operative Behandlung. In: Dermatochirurgie in Klinik und Praxis, ed. by B. Konz and G. Burg, pp. 137–144. Berlin-Heidelberg-New York: Springer 1977.

364. Pfister, R.: Die praktische Bedeutung der Fräs- und Stanzmethode für die dermatologische Praxis. Dermatologica (Basel) **111**, 25–30 (1955).

365. Pflüger, H.: Örtliche Betäubung oder Allgemeinnarkose bei plastischen Gesichtsoperationen. Aesthet. Med. **9**, 214–218 (1960).

366. Phelan, J.T., Juardo, J.: Mohs' chemosurgery technic in the management of carcinoma of the scalp. Am. J. Surg. **108**, 440–443 (1964).

367. Pick, J.F.: Surgery of Repair, Vol. I. Philadelphia, J.B. Lippincott 1949.

368. Pickrell, K.L., Georgiade, N., Adamson, J., Matton, G.: Surgical treatment of early carcinoma of the face. Postgrad. Med. **27**, 406–415 (1960).

369. Pilla, A.: Aesthetische Gesichtspunkte bei der Entfernung von Lidkarzinomen. Aesthet. Med. **11**, 139–143 (1962).

370. Pinkus, H.: Therapy of skin cancer. Clin. Med. **7**, 701–711 (1960).

371. Pirner, F.: Der variköse Symptomenkomplex. Stuttgart: Enke 1957.

372. Pitanguy, V.: Abdominal lipectomy: an approach to it through an analysis of 300 consecutive cases. Plast. Reconstr. Surg. **40**, 384–391 (1967).

373. Pitanguy, I., Treciak, H.: Operative Therapie bei Nasenspitzenläsionen. Aesthet. Med. **18**, 233–234 (1969).

374. Piulachs, P., Mir, L.: Recidivas y pseudorecidivas en al cáncer cutáneo. An. Med. Cir. (Barcelona) **46**, 111–115 (1960).

375. Plaza, F., Avello, A.: Carcinoma del labio. Acta Cancer. **5**, 49–56 (1966).

376. Pless, J., Sødergaard, W.: The effect of halothane on tissue necrosis in pedicle skin flaps in pigs. Scand. J. Plast. Reconstr. Surg. **6**, 13–15 (1972).

377. Pollack, R.S.: The surgical treatment of advanced visible cancer. In: Skin Surgery (ed. E. Epstein), 2nd ed., pp. 168–184. Philadelphia: Lea & Febiger 1962.

378. Pollock, J., Virnelli, F.R., Ryan, R.F.: Axillary hidradenitis suppurative. A simple and effective surgical technique. Plast. Reconstr. Surg. **49**, 22–27 (1972).

379. Profirov, D.: Der Röntgenkombinationsschaden bei der Nachbestrahlung des Hautkrebses. Strahlentherapie **123**, 285–289 (1964).

380. Prpić, I.: Kirurśko lijećenje malignih tumora koźe. Lijec. Vjesn. **87**, 1197–1206 (1965).

381. Pyrhönen, S., Penttinen, K.: Wart-virus antibodies and the prognosis of wart disease. Lancet **1972 II**, 1330–1332.

382. Rassner, G.: Keratoakanthom. In: Fortschr. Prakt. Dermatol. Venerol. (eds. O. Braun-Falco, D. Petzoldt), Vol. 7, pp. 52–58. Berlin-Heidelberg-New York: Springer 1973.

383. Ratzkowski, E., Hochman, A., Buchner, A., Michman, J.: Cancer of the lip. Review of 167 cases. Oncologica (Basel) **20**, 129–144 (1966).

384. Rausch, L.: Zur Behandlung von Haemangiomen und Naevi teleangiectatici. Verh. Dtsch. Dermatol. Ges., 23. Tagung, Wien 24.–27. Mai 1956. Arch. Klin. Exp. Dermatol. **206**, 123–135 (1957).

385. Rebreyoud: Zit. nach G. Scherber, Handbuch der Haut- und Geschlechtskrankheiten, Vol. XXI, S. 263 (1927). Ann. Mal. Gen.-Urin. 1898.

386. Rees, T.D.: Technical aid in blepharoplasty. Plast. Reconstr. Surg. **41**, 497–498 (1968).

387. Rees, T.D., Dupuis, Ch.C.: Baggy eyelids in young adults. Plast. Reconstr. Surg. **43**, 381–387 (1969).

388. Ress, T.D., Wood-Smith, D.: Cosmetic facial surgery. Philadelphia-London-Toronto: W.B. Saunders 1973.

389. Reichmann, W.: Funktionelle Ergebnisse nach Hautplastiken an der Hand. Aesthet. Med. **12**, 57–61 (1963).

390. Rehrmann, A., Pape, H.-D.: Die operative Behandlung der Präcancerosen. Verh.

Dtsch. Dermatol. Ges., 27. Tagung, Freiburg 29.9.–3.10. 1965. Arch. Klin. Exp. Dermatol. **227**, 819–824 (1966).

391. Rehrmann, A.: Rekonstruktion der Lippen nach Tumorentfernung. Chir. Plastica (Berl.) **3**, 222–229 (1967).

392. Reverdin, M.: Greffes épidermiques; experience faite dans le service de M. le docteur Guyon, à l'hopital Necker. Bull. Soc. Imp. Chir. (Paris), Ser. 2, **10** (1870).

393. Reymann, F.: Treatment of basal cell carcinoma of the skin with currettage. Arch. Dermatol. **103**, 623–627 (1971).

394. Reymann, F.: Treatment of basal cell carcinoma of the skin with currettage. II. A follow-up study. Arch. Dermatol. **108**, 528–531 (1973).

395. Richardson, G.S., Hanna, D.C., Gaisford, J.C.: Midline forehead flap nasal reconstructions in patients with low browlines. Plast. Reconstr. Surg. **49**, 130–133 (1972).

396. Richter, W.: Dermatologie und Chirurgie. Darstellung der Grenzgebiete für die Praxis. Leipzig: L. Voss 1936.

397. Riedel, G.: Instrumentenlehre. In: Dermatologie und Venerologie (eds. H.A. Gottron, W. Schönfeld), Vol. I/2, pp. 955–968. Stuttgart: Thieme 1962.

398. Rigg, B.M.: The dorsal nasal flap. Plast. Reconstr. Surg. **52**, 361–364 (1973).

399. Rigg, B.M.: Axillary hyperhidrosis. Plast. Reconstr. Surg. **59**, 334–346 (1977).

400. Robbins, T.H.: The "crown" excision of facial skin lesions. Plast. Reconstr. Surg. **57**, 251–254 (1976).

401. Robinson, D.W.: Surgical problems in the excision and repair of radiated tissue. Plast. Reconstr. Surg. **55**, 41–49 (1975).

402. Röckl, U., Schubert, E.: Fascitis nodularis pseudosarcomatosa. Hautarzt **22**, 150–153 (1971).

403. Rook, A.: Disorders of the connective tissue. In: Textbook of Dermatology (ed. A. Rook, D.S. Wilkinson, F.J.G. Ebling) 2nd ed., Vol. 2, pp. 1458–1495. Oxford-London-Edinburgh-Melbourne: Blackwell 1972.

404. Rook, A., Wilkinson, D.S.: The principles of diagnosis. In: Textbook of Dermatology (ed. A. Rook, D.S. Wilkinson, F.J.G. Ebling) 2nd ed., Vol. 1, pp. 37–90. Oxford-London-Edinburgh-Melbourne: Blackwell 1972.

405. Rowley, M.J., Heller, C.G.: The testicular biopsy: Surgical procedure, fixation and staining technics. Fertil. Steril. **17**, 177–186 (1966).

406. Saegesser, M.: Spezielle chirurgische Therapie, 8th ed. Bern-Stuttgart-Vienna: Huber

407. Salfeld, K.: Hyperhidrosis axillaris und Hidradenitis suppurativa. In: Dermatochirurgie in Klinik und Praxis, (ed. B. Konz, G. Burg), pp. 171–177. Berlin-Heidelberg-New York: Springer 1977.

408. Santler, R., Freilinger, G.: Operative Tumorbehandlung in der Dermatologie.—Verh. Dtsch. Dermatol. Ges., 29. Tagung, Berlin 29.9.–2.10. 1971. Arch. Dermatol. Forsch. **244**, 418–420 (1972).

409. Sarnat, B.G.: Facial plastic surgery. In: Skin Surgery (ed. E. Epstein), 2nd ed., pp. 127–167. Philadelphia: Lea & Febiger 1962.

410. Savenero-Roselli: Plastic surgery in cancer of the face and the neck. In: Andina, F., Plastic Surgery of Head and Neck Tumours. Amsterdam: Excerpta Medica Foundation 1965.

411. Schedel, F.: Plastische Chirurgie bei malignen Tumoren. Chirurg **36**, 109–113 (1965).

412. Scherber, G.: Phimose und Paraphimose. In: J. Jadassohn, Handbuch der Haut- und Geschlechtskrankheiten, Vol. XXI. Berlin: Springer 1927.

413. Schettler, D.: Oberkiefergeschwülste. Diagnostik **6**, 760–764 (1973).

414. Schiller, F., Beetz, D.: Aesthetische und klinische Gesichtspunkte bei Tätowierungen heute. Aesthest. Med. **17**, 143–150 (1968).

415. Schlenger, T.: Präcancerosen auf Röntgenhaut. — Sitzung der Vereinigung Düsseldorfer Dermatologen. Zentralbl. Haut- u. Geschl.-Kr. **121**, 167 (1966).

416. Schlockermann, F.W.: Zur Therapie der Onychomykosen. Hautarzt **8**, 270–271 (1957).

417. Schmid, E.: Die Indikationen und Möglichkeiten kosmetisch-operativer Eingriffe im Gesicht (I). Therapiewoche **11**, 63–71 (1960).

418. Schmid, E.: Sekundärplastik nach Verbrennungsschäden der Lippen. Chir. Plastica (Berl.) **1**, 143–148 (1966).

419. Schmid, E.: Neue Möglichkeiten in der plastischen Chirurgie durch subdermale Implantationen von Composite grafts und von Millipore. Chir. Plastica (Berl.) **5**, 246–253 (1968).

420. Schmid, M.A.: Die freie Verpflanzung flächenförmiger Hautlappen. Vorträge aus der prakt. Chir., Heft 73. Stuttgart: Enke 1965.

421. Schmidt-Tintemann, U.: Sekundärplastische Maßnahmen nach Verbrennung im Bereich der unteren Gesichtshälfte und des Halses. Chir. Plastica (Berl.) **1**, 149–153 (1966).

tischen Chirurgie. Berlin-Heidelberg-New York: Springer 1972.

423. Schmiedt, E., Elsässer, E.: Operative Maßnahmen bei Fertilitätsstörungen. Fortschr. prakt. Dermatol. Venerol. (eds. O. Braun-Falco, D. Petzoldt), Vol. 7, pp. 164–173. Berlin-Heidelberg-New York: Springer 1973.

424. Schneider, W.: Kritisches zur Nachbestrahlung maligner Tumoren. Strahlentherapie **84**, 284–296 (1951).

425. Schneider, W.: Zur Differentialdiagnose der grau-braun-blauschwarzen ,,Tumoren''. Diagnostik 7, 215–219 (1974).

426. Schnyder, U.W., Keller, R.: Zur Klinik und Histologie der Angiome. III. Mitteilung: Zur Histologie und Pathogenese der senilen Angiome. Arch. Dermatol. Syph. (Berl.) **198**, 333–342 (1955).

427. Schnyder, U.W.: Zur Klinik und Histologie der Angiome. IV. Mitteilung: Die planotuberösen und tubero-nodösen Angiome des Kleinkindes. Arch. Klin. Exp. Dermatol. **204**, 457–471 (1957).

428. Schnyder, U.W.: Zur Indikation und Technik der Probeexzision bei Hautkrankheiten. Praxis **51**, 922–924 (1961).

429. Schnyder, U.W., Goos, M., Riderer, K.: Superficial spreading melanoma. Dtsch. Med. Wochenschr. **98**, 1899–1900 (1973).

430. Schöberlin, W.: Bedeutung und Häufigkeit von Phimose und Smegma. Münch. Med. Wochenschr. **108**, 373–377 (1966).

431. Schoop, W.: Angiologie-Fibel. Stuttgart: G. Thieme 1967.

432. Schraffordt Koops, H.: Melanoblastoma malignum cutis van de extremiteiten regionale perfusie en recidief. Assen: Van Gorcum K. Comp. 1973.

433. Schreus, H.T.: Hochtouriges Schleifen der Haut (Ein neues Behandlungsverfahren). Z. Hautkr. **8**, 151–156 (1950).

434. Schreus, H.Th.: Hochtouriges Schleifen der Haut (Demonstration). Verh. Dtsch. Dermatol. Ges., 21. Tagung, Heidelberg 6.–9.9. 1949; Arch. Dermatol. Syph. (Berl.) **191**, 678–679 (1950).

435. Schreus, H.T.: Chlorzinkschnellätzung des Epithelioms. Ein Beitrag zur Chemochirurgie. Hautarzt **2**, 317–319 (1951).

436. Schreus, H.T.: Weitere Erfahrungen mit hochtourigem Schleifen der Haut. In: Arztgliche Kosmetik, Heft 1. Heidelberg: Hüthig 1955.

437. Schreus, H.T.: Schleifen und Fräsen der Haut. In: Ärztliche Kosmetik, Heft 2. Heidelberg: Hüthig 1956.

438. Schreus, H.Th.: Diskussionsbemerkung zu:

sichtskorrekturen durch hochtourige Glättungsverfahren. Aesthet. Med. **13**, 260 (1964).

439. Schröder, F.: Zur Verwendung gestielter Lappen in der Plastischen Chirurgie des Kiefer-Gesichtsbereiches. Experimentelle Untersuchungen und klinische Beobachtungen. Habil.-Schr. Hamburg 1960.

440. Schröder, F.: Bildung von Gesichtschautlappen unter besonderer Berücksichtigung der Gefäßversorgung nach Entfernung von Geisichtstumoren. Chir. Plastica (Berl.) **3**, 184–187 (1967).

441. Schröder, F.: Deckung von Gesichtsdefekten nach tumoroperationen beim Patienten höheren Alters. Chir. Plastica (Berl.) **5**, 152–162 (1968).

442. Schrudde, J.: Die Deckung von Hautdefekten durch gestielte Lappenplastik. Aesthet. Med. **12**, 166–173 (1963).

443. Schrudde, J.: Primary soft tissue plastic operations following removal of malignant tumours. In: Andina, F., Plastic surgery of head and neck tumours. Int. Congress Series No. 98. Amsterdam: Excerpta Medica Foundation 1965.

444. Schuchardt, K.: Die Rundstiellappen in der Wiederherstellungschirurgie des Gesichts-Kieferbereichs. Leipzig: Thieme 1944.

445. Schuchardt, K.: Ausgewählte Kapitel aus der Wiederherstellungschirurgie des Gesichts unter besonderer Berücksichtigung der Augenlider und der Orbita. In: R. Thiel, Ophthalmologische Operationslehre, Vol. 4. Leipzig: Thieme 1950.

446. Schuchardt, K.: Operationen an Kopf und Wirbelsäule. In: Bier-Braun-Kümmel, Operationen am Gesichtsteil des Kopfes, 7th ed. Vol. II. Leipzig: J.A. Barth 1954.

447. Schuchardt, K.: Plastische Operationen im Mund- und Kieferbereich. In: Zahn-Mund-Kieferheilkunde (eds. K. Häupl, W. Meyer, K. Schuchardt), Vol. III, part 2. Munich-Berlin: Urban & Schwarzenberg 1959.

448. Schuchardt, K.: Grundsätzliches zur primären und sekundären Defektdeckung nach der Operation von gutartigen und bösartigen Gesichtstumoren. Chir. Plastica (Berl.) **3**, 180–183 (1967).

449. Schuchardt, K.: Operationen an Kopf und Wirbelsäule. In: Bier-Braun-Kümmel, Operationen am Gesichtsteil des Kopfes, 8th ed., Vol. 2. Leipzig: J.A. Barth 1970.

450. Schuermann, H.: Krankheiten der Mundschleimhaut und der Lippen, 2. Aufl. Munich-Berlin: Urban & Schwarzenberg 1958.

451. Schulte-Steinberg, O.: Zwischenfälle bei der Lokalanaesthesie. Diagnostik **6**, 724–728

452. Schulz, K.A.: Über eine neue Verödungs-
therapie der Akne conglobata und cys-
tischen Akne vulgaris. Z. Hautkr. **49**, 65–68
(1974).

453. Schwenzer, N.: Geschwülste im Lippen-
und Gesichtsbereich. Diagnostik **6**, 750–754
(1973).

454. Schwenzer, N.: Das menschliche Gesicht
— operative Herstellung und Korrektur.
Dtsch. Ärztebl. **70**, 3386–3391 (1973).

455. Seemen, H.von: Operative Behandlung
schwerer Strahlenschädigungen. Langen-
becks Arch. Klin. Chir. **270**, 363–366,
(1951).

456. von Seemen, H., Antoine, L.: Plastische
Chirurgie und Kosmetik. Munich: Urban
& Schwarzenberg 1958.

457. Serćer, A., Mündnich, K.: Plastische Operationen an der Nase und an der Ohrmuschel. Stuttgart: Thieme 1962.

458 Shah, J.P., Goldsmith, H.S.: Incontinuity
versus discontinuous lymph node dissection
for malignant melanoma. Cancer (Philad.)
26, 610–614 (1970).

459. Sigg, K.,: Ulcus cruris, Varicen und Throm-
bose. Berlin-Heidelberg-New York: Springer 1976.

460. Skoog, T.: Die chirurgische Behandlung
von Verbrennungen der Lider und Augen-
brauen. Chir. Plastica (Berl.) **1**, 126–134
(1966).

461. Smith, F.: Plastic and Reconstructive Surgery—a Manual of Management. Philadelphia: Saunders 1950.

462. Spiessl, B.: Möglichkeiten der Schnittführung zur en-block-Resektion der Mundhöhle und des Gesichts. Dtsch. Zahn-,
Mund-Kieferheilkd. **43**, 190–200 (1964).

463. Spira, M., Hardy, S.B.: Vermilionectomy.
Plast. Reconstr. Surg. **33**, 39–46 (1964).

464. Spira, M.: Lower blepharoplasty—a clinical
study. Plast. Reconstr. Surg. **59**, 35–38
(1977).

465. Steigleder, G.K.: Grundsätzliches zur his-
tologischen Technik in der Dermatologie.
In: Dermatologie und Venerologie (eds.
H.A. Gottron, W. Schönfeld). Stuttgart:
Thieme 1961.)

466. Steigleder, G.K.: Die Präcancerosen in
moderner Sicht. Hautarzt **14**, 87–94 (1963).

467. Steigleder, G.K.: Diagnostische Möglichkeiten der Dermatohistopathologie.
Hautarzt **19**, 447–451 (1968).

468. Steigleder, G.K.: Dermatologie und Venerologie für Ärzte und Studenten. 2nd Ed.
Stuttgart: Thieme 1975.

469. Steigleder, G.K., Gartmann, H.: Malignes
Melanom: Hinweise zur Diagnostik für die
Praxis. Diagnostik **7**, 220–226 (1974).

470. Steinacher, J.: Zur Behandlung der Böller-
schuβverletzungen. Cosmetologie **19**, 15–17
(1970).

471. Stühmer, A.: Demonstration über die Technik der Anwendung von Stanzen und Fräsen. Dritte Dermatologische Woche, Freiburg i.Br. 1953.

472. Sulzberger, M.B., Witten, V.H.: Why der-
matologic surgery? In: Skin Surgery (ed. E.
Epstein), 2nd ed., pp. 15–22. Philadelphia:
Lea & Febiger 1962.

473. Sundell, B., Gylling, U., Soivio, A.I.:
Treatment of basal cell carcinoma by plastic
surgery. Acta Chir. Scand. **131**, 249–253
(1966).

474. Sutton, R.: Diseases of the Skin, 11th ed.
St. Louis: C.V. Mosby 1956.

475. Thiersch, C.: Über Hautverpflanzung. —
Verh. Dtsch. Ges. Chir., 15. Kongress,
7.–10.4. 1886. Suppl. to Zentralbl. Chir. **13**,
17–18 (1886).

476. Thöne, A.W.: Die Behandlung der Verruca
senilis und der Keratosis praecancerosa.
Hautarzt **10**, 468–471 (1959).

477. Trauner, R.: Plastiken bei Gesichtshäman-
giomen. Aesthet. Med. **10**, 69–78 (1961).

478. Trauner, R.: Kiefer- und Gesichtschirurgie.
Munich-Berlin-Vienna: Urbab & Schwarzenberg 1973.

479. Trautmann, A.C., Converse, J.M., Smith,
B.: Plastic and Reconstructive Surgery of
the Eye and Adnexa. Washington: Butter-
worths 1962.

480. Tritsch, H.: Behandlung von Bestrahlungs-
folgen der Haut. Chir. Praxis **8**, 129–138
(1964).

481. Tromovitsch, T.A.: Skin cancer. Treatment
by curettage and desiccation. Calif. Med.
103, 107–108 (1965).

482. Tromovitsch, T.A., Beirne, G., Beirne, C.:
Cancer chemosurgery (Mohs technique).
The "chemo-check". Arch. Dermatol. **92**,
291–292 (1965).

483. Villoria, J.M.F.: A new method of elonga-
tion of the corner of the mouth. Plast. Reconstr. Surg. **49**, 52–55 (1972).

484. Vogt, H., Neumann, L.: Operative Behandlung der männlichen Glatze. Hautarzt **19**,
518–520 (1968).

485. Vonkennel, J., Fiebig, M.: Kosmetisch Stö-
rende Erkrankungen der Haut einschließ-
lich der Therapie. In: Dermatologie und
Venerologie (eds. H.A. Gottron, W. Schönfeld), Vol. II, Part 1, pp. 287–312. Stuttgart:
Thieme 1958.

486. Walter, C.: Hinweise auf Möglichkeiten der plastisch-chirurgischen Versorgung von Krankheits- oder Unfallfolgen im Gesicht. Aesthet. Med. **17**, 87–94 (1968).

487. Walter, C.: Plastisch-chirurgische Gesichtspunkte der primären Wundversorgung und der sekundären Narbenkorrektur im Gesichts und Halsbereich. Aesthet. Med. **18**, 73–84 (1969).

488. Walter, C.: Chirurgie. Cosmetologica **19**, 171–178 (1970).

489. Wanebo, H.W., Fortner, J.G., Woodruff, J., MacLean, B., Binkowski, E.: Selection of the optimum surgical treatment of stage I melanoma by depth of microinvasion. Ann. Surg. **182**, 302–315 (1975).

490. Wanebo, H.W., Woodruff, J., Fortner, J.G.: Malignant melanoma of the extremities: a clinicopathologic study using levels of invasion (microstage). Cancer **35**, 666–676 (1975).

491. Wassmund, M.: Lehrbuch der praktischen Chirurgie des Mundes und der Kiefer. Leipzig: H. Meusser 1935, 1939.

492. Weaver, P.C., Copeman, P.W.M.: Simple surgery for axillary hyperhidrosis, two cases. Proc. Roy. Soc. Med. **64**, 607–608 (1971).

493. Wegener, E.H.: Wann verspricht die Epicraniotomie einen Erfolg und was ist bei der Operationstechnik zu beachten? Aesthet. Med. **10**, 123–126 (1961).

494. Weidner, F., Hornstein, O.P.: Das Problem der regionalen Lymphknotenmetastasierung bei malignen Melanomen. Arch. Dermatol. Forsch. **245**, 50–62 (1972).

495. Weissleder, H., Pfannenstiel, P.: Endolymphatische Metastasentherapie mit Radioisotopen beim malignen Melanom. — Verh. Dtsch. Dermat. Ges., 29. Tagung, Berlin 29.9.–2.10.1971. Arch. Derm. Forsch. **244**, 245–250 (1972).

496. Werner, H.: Die Indikation zur Strahlentherapie unter aesthetischem Gesichtspunkt. Aesthet. Med. **15**, 34–43 (1966).

497. Wernsdörfer, R.: Carcinome der Ohrmuschel. Bericht über 170 Fälle. Z. Hautkr. **42**, 303–308 (1967).

498. Widmaier, W.: Funktionelle und kosmetische Mißerfolge bei Sekundäroperationen nach Verbrennungen des Gesichtes und des Halses infolge mangelhafter Operationsplanung. Chir. Plastica (Berl.) **1**, 163–169 (1966).

499. Wiedemann, G.: Erfahrungen mit der externen Colchicin-Behandlung in der Dermatologie. — Verh. Dtsch. Dermatol. Ges., 23. Tagung, Vienna, 24.–27.5.1956. Arch. Klin. Exp. Dermatol. **206**, 686–689 (1957).

500. Wiendl, H.-J.: Die chirurgische Behandlung von Strahlenulcera. Chir. Plastica (Berl.) **6**, 221–234 (1969).

501. Wilkinson, D.S.: Physical and surgical procedures. In: Textbook of Dermatology (eds. A. Rook, Wilkinson, D.S., Ebling. F.J.G.), 2nd ed., Vol. 2, pp. 2088–2104. Oxford-London-Edinburgh-Melbourne: Blackwell 1972.

502. Winkelmann, M.: Zur chirurgischen Behandlung der Elephantiasis der Extremitäten. Med. Kosmetik **6**, 225–233 (1957).

503. Wiskemann, A.: Zur Melanomentstehung durch chronische Lichteinwirkung. Hautarzt **25**, 20–22 (1974).

504. Wolfe, J.R.: A new method for performing plastic operations. Brit. Med. J. **1875II**, 360.

505. Woolf, R.M., Broadbent, T.R.: The four-flap Z-plasty. Plast. Reconstr. Surg. **49**, 48–51 (1972).

506. Wullstein, H.L.: Chirurgische Zusammenarbeit im ,,Kopfbereich''. Dtsch. Ärztebl. **70**, 3134–3137 (1973).

507. Zacarian, S.A.: Cryosurgery of Tumors of the Skin and Oral Cavity. Springfield, Ill.: C.C Thomas 1973.

508. Zehm, S.: Primär plastische Versorgung von Hautdefekten an Hals und Kiefer unter besonderer Berücksichtigung des gestielten Brusthautlappens. Chir. Plastica (Berl.) **3**, 256–263 (1967).

509. Ziegenbalg, H.: Therapie der Strahlenschäden der Haut. Aesthet. Med. **14**, 74–84 (1965).

510. Ziemann, S.A.: Das Lymphödem. Stuttgart: Hippokrates 1964.

511. Zile, W.N. van: Early carcinoma of the lip: diagnosis and treatment. J. Oral. Surg. **23**, 50–59 (1965).

512. Zoltan, J.: Die plastische Deckung von Defekten nach Excision von Strahlenschäden der Haut. Chir. Plastica (Berl.) **2**, 1–11 (1966).

513. Zwicker, M.: Beitrag zur operativen Behandlung der Elephantiasis. Med. Kosmetik **6**, 220–225 (1957).

514. Zwinggi, F.: Beingeschwüre, Varizen und Thrombosen. Bern: Huber 1964.

Index

A

Abdomen, sagging, rehabilitation of, 84–85
Acanthokeratoma, 11
Acanthoma, clear cell, 5
Acne abscedens, 25–26
Acne conglobata, 25
Acne keloid, 25
Acne pustules, 27
Actinic keratosis, 3, 9
Actinic leukoplakia, 9
Actinomyces, diseases due to, 27
Adenoma, sebaceous gland, 6, 19
Advancement flap technique, 44
  see also Lateral advancement flap technique
  for auricle, 79–80
  for cheeks, 75
  for chin defect, 81
  for eyelids, 70–71
  for temporal region, 54, 56
Ala nasi
  composite graft for, 64
  rotation flap technique for, 59–61
Anesthesia
  procedures for, 38–40
  types of, 38–40
Angiokeratoma, 21
  neviforme, 21
Angiokeratoma akroasphyticum Mibelli, 21
Angiokeratoma inpunctiformae scroti s. vulvae
  Fordyce, 21
Angioleiomyoma, 22
Angiolipoma, 20
Angioma
  eruptive, 20–21
  thrombosed, 21
Angioma senile, 21
Angiomyoneuroma, 22
Antimicrobial powder, 38
Apocrine cystadenoma, 6

Armpit,
  see Axilla
Arsenic keratosis, 8
Arteriosclerotic gangrene, of leg, 30
Atheroma, 7, 13
Atraumatic epidermal cysts, 7
Atropine, 35
Auricle
  advancement flap technique for, 79
  caudal advancement flap technique for, 7
  other flap techniques for, 75–83
  partial amputation of, 76
  reduction plasty of, 76, 79
  rotation flap technique for, 78–80
  transposition flap technique for, 78–80
  triangular excision for, 78
Autologous skin transplants, 34
Axilla, flap technique for, 85–86
Axillary hyperhidrosis, 31–32
  surgical therapy for, 86–87

B

Baggy eyelids, correction of, 72–75
  see also Eyelids
Balanitis plasmocellularis, 9
Balanoposthitis, 9
Bartholinitis, 26
Basal amelanotic nevus, 6
Basal cell carcinoma, 3, 5–6, 9–13, 17–21
  morphea-like, 33–34
  nevoid, 13
  nodular forms of, 34
  retroauricular, 34
Basal cell epithelioma, 12
Basal cell nevus syndrome, 13
Basal cell papilloma, 3–5, 9, 21
Basalioma, *see* Basal cell carcinoma
Besnier-Boeck-Schaumann disease, 27

Biopsy, skin, 42
Blackheads, removal of, 26
Blepharochalasis, 32
Blepharoplasty, 72–77
Bowen's disease, 3, 8–10, 16, 33, 40, 87
Burns and scalding, 30–31
   chemical, 31
Burow's triangle, 45, 46

C

Callosities, 30
Candidiasis, 9
Cantharidin blistering method, 5
Capillary hemangioma, 21–22
Carcinoid mucosal papillomatosis, 11
Carcinomas, 10–12
   basal cell, *see* Basal cell carcinoma
   squamous cell, *see* Squamous cell carcinoma
Caudal advancement flap technique, 53–54, 77
   for nose, 60
Caudal rotation flap technique, for temporal
   region, 54–55
Cavernous hemangioma, 22
Cellulitis, dissecting of the scalp, 25, 81
Cheek
   dermatosurgery for, 75
   port wine stain of, 127
Cheilitis abrasiva precancerosa (Manganotti), 9
Cheilitis granulomatosa, 27
   surgical therapy for, 69
Chemical burns, 31
Chemosurgery, 49
   avoidance of, 4
Chessboard graft, 91
Chin defect
   advancement flap technique for, 81
   rotation flap technique for, 81–82
Chondrodermatitis nodularis helicis chronica, 8
Cicatricial post-inflammatory states, 27–30
Circumcision, 86
Clear cell acanthoma, 5
Coagulation, in electrosurgery, 48
Cockett operation, 91–92
Columella nasi reconstruction technique, 62
Conduction anesthesia, 39–40
Condyloma acuminatum, 5
Connective tissues
   benign tumors of, 17–19
   pseudotumors of, 17–19
   semimalignant and malignant tumors of, 19
Continuous intradermic sutures, in
   dermatosurgery, 41–42
Corial foreign body intrusions, 30
Cornu cutaneum, 8

Cosmetic disorders, 31–32
Cosmetic surgery, 32
Cranial advancement flap technique, for nose,
   59–60
Cutaneous horn, 8
Cutaneous veins, varicose dilations of, 28–29
Cutis hyperelastica, 24
Cutis laxa, 24
Cylindroma, 6
Cysts, 6–7
   atraumatic epidermal, 7
   of jaw, 13
   traumatic epithelial, 30

D

Dehungsplastik, 34, 38, 86
   described, 43
   for hands and feet, 92
   for sagging abdomen, 84
Dental skin fistulas, 27
Dermabrasion, 5, 47–48
   low-speed, 3
   for hands and feet, 92
Dermal cylindroma, 13
Dermatitis perianalis fistulosa, 25
Dermatofibroma lenticulare Schreus, 17
Dermatofibrosarcoma protuberans, 19
Dermatology, surgical indications in, 3–32
   see also Dermatosurgery
Dermatopathy, of leg, 29
Dermatosurgery
   anatomic features in, 36
   anesthesia in, 38–40
   basic principles of, 33–49
   combination of flap techniques, 46
   conduction anesthesia and, 39–40
   continuous intradermic sutures in, 41–42
   dermabrasion in, 47–48
   electrosurgery in, 48
   flaps and grafts from other body areas in,
     46–47
   general anesthesia in, 40
   incision techniques in, 41
   interrupted sutures in, 41
   for lips, 64–70
   local anesthesia in, 39
   marginal wall anesthesia in, 39
   mattress sutures in, 41
   pre- and postoperative care in, 35, 37–38
   requirements and considerations in, 33–34
   skin biopsy in, 42
   special regional anesthesia procedures in, 40
   special techniques for different body regions
     in, 51–92

superextension in, 37
surgical instruments in, 34–35
surgical techniques in, 42–46
suture removal in, 42
Desmoid tumor, 19
Dessication, in electrosurgery, 48
Dorsal incision, for paraphimosis, 86
Dorsal rotation flap technique, for temporal region, 54
Double lateral advancement technique, for nose, 60
Double transposition flap technique, 58
Double rotation flap technique
  for scalp, 51
  for trunk, 83
Dubreuilh's disease, 15–16
Dubreuilh's melanoma, 16
  see also Lentigo maligna
Dupuytren's contracture, 24
Dysplasias, 24

E

Eccrine poroma, 6
Eccrine spiradenoma, 6
Eczema, of nipple aerola, 11
Electrodesiccation, 4
Electrosurgery, 48
Electrotomy, 48
Elephantiasis nostras, 29
Elliptical excision, with primary wound closure, 42–43
Epidermal cysts, 7
  atraumatic, 7
  traumatic, 7
Epidermal hyperplasia, reactive, 10
Epidermal nevi, rare, 5
Epidermoid cysts, 7
Epithelioma, 6
  adenoides cysticum, 6
  calcifying, 6
  Malherbe's, 6
Epithelioma adenoides cysticum Brooke, 13
Epithelioma planum et cicatricans, 12
Eruptive angioma, 20
Erythroplasia of Queyrat, 9, 87
Extremities, transposition flap technique for, 90
Eyelids
  advancement flap technique for, 70–71
  baggy, 72–75, 130
  blepharoplasty of, 72–75
  rotation flap technique for, 71–72
  surgical repair of, 70–75
  transposition flap technique for, 71–72

F

Fabry's disease, 21
Facial surgery, anatomic features in, 36
Fasciitis nodularis, 19
Fat hernias, blepharoplasty and, 73
Fatty tissue, tumors of, 20
Female genital region, dermatosurgery of, 90
Fibroplasia, nontumorous, 19
Fibroses, 24
Fifth phacomatosis, 13
Fig wart, 5
Finger
  radiation ulcer of, 41
  verruca vulgaris of, 42
Flaps
  for temporal region, 53–55
  tubed pedicled, 47
  types of, 44–46
Flap techniques
  basic principles, 44–47
  for auricle, pre- and postauricular regions, 75–83
  cranial advancement, 59
  double transposition, 58
  for forehead, 55–56
  lateral advancement, 58–59
  for nose, 57–64
Follicle retention cysts, 7, 13, 27
Folliculitis keloidalis, 25
Folliculitis nuchae sclerotisans, 25
  see Cellulitis
Forehead
  flap techniques for, 55–56
  wrinkles in, 32
Foreign bodies, lesions due to, 30
Foreign body granuloma, 30
Freckles, 14
Free skin grafting, 46–47
  for hands and feet, 92
  for nose, 63
  for temporal region, 54–55
  for trunk, 83–84
Fulguration, in electrosurgery, 48
Full-thickness skin grafts, 46
  for scalp, 52
Functional disorders, 31–32

G

Galuschka's solution, 26
Gangrene, of leg, 30
General anesthesia, in dermatosurgery, 40
Glomangioma, 22
Glomus tumor, multiple familial, 22

Grafts, 46–47
  free skin, 46
  full thickness skin, 46
  in leg ulcer, 29–30
  punch, 47
  split-thickness skin, 29, 47, 90–91
Granular cell myoblastoma, 22
Granuloma, 20
  "talcum," 38
Granuloma pediculatum, 20
Granuloma "pyogenicum," 20
Griseofulvin therapy, 32

H

Hair follicle nevus, 6
Hair follicles, inflammations originating from, 25
Hairy mole, 15
Hairy nevus, 137
Halo nevus, Sutton's, 14
Hammer nose, 6
Hands and feet, dermatosurgery of, 92
Hemangioendothelioma, 23
Hemangioma
  capillary, 21–22
  cavernous, 22
Hemangioma simplex, 21
Hemangiopericytoma, 23
Hemangiosarcoma, 23
Hemoblastoses, malignant, 20
Hidradenectomy, 86
Hidradenitis suppurativa, 26
Histocytoma, 19–21
Hydradenoma papilliferum, 6
Hyperhidrosis axillary, 31–32, 86–87
  elliptical excision for, 87
Hyperplasias of the skin, 24
Hypertrophic scars, 19

I

Incision techniques, in dermatosurgery, 41
Induratio penis plastica, 24
Internal carcinomas, skin metastases of, 11
  see also Basal cell carcinoma; Squamous cell carcinoma
Island flap technique, 45–46, 62

J

Juvenile melanoma, 15
Juvenile palmoplantar fibrosis, 24
Juvenile xanthogranuloma, 18
Juvenile xanthoma, 18

K

Kaposi's sarcoma, 23
Keloid, 18, 30
Keratoacanthoma, 10–11, 14, 21, 25
Keratoma solare, 7–8
Keratosis
  actinic, 7
  arsenic, 8
  senilis, 7
  solar, 7–8, 30
  tar and oil, 8
Kraurosis vulvae, 90

L

Lateral advancement flap technique, 58–59
Leg
  arteriosclerotic and diabetic gangrene of, 30
  dermatopathy of, 29
Leg ulcer, 29–30
  surgical therapy for, 90–92
Leiomyoma, 22
Leishmaniasis, 27
Lentigo, 14
Lentigo maligna, 15–16, 33
Lentigo maligna melanoma, 16
Lentigo senilis, 14, 16
Leukoplakia, 9, 33
Lichen sclerosus et atrophicans, 9–10
Lip
  cancer of, 64
  congenital dimple of, 24
  dermatosurgery of, 64–70
  lower, see Lower lip
  squamous cell carcinoma of, 23
  triangular excision in, 65–66
  vermilionectomy for, 64–65
Lipoma, 20
Lipomatosis dolorosa, 20
Liquid nitrogen, 4
Liver stars, 21
Lower lip
  see also Lip
  advancement flap techniques for, 66
  repair of, 66–67, 69
  transposition flap technique for, 67–68
  VY-flap technique for, 62
Lupus vulgaris, 26, 33
Lymphadenosis cutis benigna Baefverstedt, 20
Lymphangiomas, 22–23
Lymphangioplasty, 88
Lymphocytoma cutis, 20
Lymphogranulomatosis, malignant, 20
Lymphomas, malignant, 20

M

Male genital region, flap techniques for, 86–89
  see also Penis
Malherbe's epithelioma, 6
Malignant melanoma, 16–17, 21
Malignant neogenesis, prevention of, 33–34
Mandible defect, rotation flap technique for, 82
Mastocytoma faciale, 20
Mattress sutures, 41
Melanoma, 3
  juvenile, 15
  lentigo maligna, 16
  malignant, 3, 16–17, 21
  superficial spreading, 16
Melanophacomatosis, 15
Melkersson-Rosenthal syndrome, 69
Mesh graft, 91
Milia, 7
Minor's sweat test, 31
Moles, 14
  hairy, 15
Molluscum contagiosum, 5
Molluscum pseudocarcinomatosum, 11
Molluscum sebaceum, 11
Morbus Bowen, 10
Mouth, plastic surgery for widening of, 68
Multiple Z flaps, for extremities, 90–92
Muscle systems, benign tumors of, 20–21
Mycoses, deep, 27

N

Nails
  extraction of, 92
  lesions of, 32
Necrotizing perifolliculitis, 25
Nerves and nerve sheaths, tumors of, 24
Neurilemmona, 24
Neurocutaneous melanoblastosis, 15
Neurofibroma, 24
Neurofibromatosis, 24
Neurofibrosarcoma, 24
Nevi, *see* Nevus
Nevoid basal cell carcinoma, 13
Nevoxanthoendothelioma, 18
Nevoxanthoma, 18
Nevus
  epidermal, 5
  hairy, 37
  spider, 21
Nevus araneus, 21
Nevus coeruleus, 15
Nevus comedonicus, 6
Nevus flammeus, 23

Nevus flammeus medialis, 23
Nevus papillomatosus, 14
Nevus pigmentosus, 6, 13–15, 21
Nevus pilosus, 15
Nevus sebaceus, 5
Nevus verrucosus, 5
Nevus vinosus, 23
Nipple, Paget's disease of, 10
Nitric acid, 4
Nodular malignant melanoma, 16–17
Nodular subepidermal fibrosis Michelson, 17
Nodulus cutaneous Arning-Lewandrowsky, 17
Nose
  caudal advancement flap technique for, 60
  columella nasi reconstruct technique for, 62
  composite grafts for, 62
  cranial advancement flap technique for, 60
  double lateral advancement flap technique
    for, 60
  flap techniques for, 56–64
  free skin grafting for, 63
  rhinophyma therapy, 63–64
  rotation flap technique, 59–61
  tunnel flap technique for, 61–62
  Z-flap technique for, 63

O

Odoriferous glands, inflammations originating
    in, 26
Oil keratoses, 8
Onchomycoses, 32
Oral florid papillomatosis, 11–12

P

Pachydermia vegetans, 29
Paget's disease, 10
Palmoplantar fibrosis, 24
Palmoplantar keratoses, 8
Paltauf-Sternberg-Hodgkin
    lymphogranulomatosis, 20
Papilloma, virus, *see* Virus papilloma
Papillomatosis, oral florid, 11–12
Papillomatosis cutis, 29
Papillomatosis cutis carcinoides Gottron, 11
Papillomatous nevus pigmentosus, 3
Paraphimosis, 27, 86
Penis
  anesthesia of, 40
  amputation of, 88
  circumcision of, 86
  elephantiasis of, 88
  free skin grafting technique for, 88
  lymphangioplasty and, 88–89

pedicled flap technique for glans, 87–88
phimosis correction, 87
Perifolliculitis capitis abscedens et suffodiens, 27
    deep necrotizing, 25
Phacomatosis Bourneville-Pringle, 19
Phimosis, 27, 39
Phimosis correction, 87
Pigmented mole, 14
Pigment-producing cells
    benign tumors of, 14
    premalignant and malignant neogenesis in, 15–17
Pilomatrixoma, 6
Plantar wart, 4–5
Pneumothorax, in anesthesia, 40
Postthrombotic syndrome, 27–30
Potato nose, 6
Pre- and postoperative care, 35, 37–38
Precanceroses, 7–10
Premalignant fibroepithelial tumor, 13
Premalignant melanosis Dubreuilh, 15–16
Prepuce, strictures of, 27
Prickle cell carcinoma, 10
Primary wound closure, 42–43
Proliferative subcutaneous fasciitis, 19
Pseudocancerous lesions, 11–12
Pseudocarcinomous hyperplasia, 11
Pseudosarcomatous fasciitis, 19
Pseudotumors, of connective tissues, 17–19
Pseudoxanthoma elasticum, 24
Psyquil, 37
Punch grafts, 47
Pyodermia fistulans sinifica, 25–26

Q

Queyrat, erythroplasia of, 9, 87

R

Radiation therapy, avoidance of, 4
Radiodermatitis, 9
Recklinghausen's neurofibrosis, 24
Regional flaps, 44–46
Relaxed skin tension lines, 35
Reticulosarcomatosis, 20
Reverdin's punch graft, 29, 90–91
Rhinophyma, 6, 63–64
Roentgenism, 9
Rotation flap technique, 45–46
    for ala nasi defects, 60–61
    for axilla, 85
    for auricle, 78–80

for cheeks, 75
for chin defect, 81–82
for eyelids, 71–72
for forehead, 56
free skin graft and, 51–52
for lower eyelid, 74
for mandible defect, 82
for scalp, 51
for throat, 82
for trunk, 83

S

Sagging abdomen, rehabilitation of, 84–85
Salicylic acid plaster, 4
Sarcoidosis, 27
Scalding and burns, 30–31
Scalp
    flap techniques for, 51–53
    full thickness skin graft for, 52
    relaxation of, 52–53
    surgery for, 52–53
    transplantation of multiple punch biopsies of, 52
Sclerosing angioma Gross-Wolbach, 18
Scrofulderma, 27
Scrotal area
    repairs in, 88
    testicular biopsy and, 89
Sebaceous gland adenoma, 6
Sebaceous gland hyperplasia, 5–6
Sebaceous gland, inflammations originating from, 25
Seborrheic keratosis, 3–4
Senile angiectasia, 21
Senile sebaceous gland hyperplasia, 6
Shock therapy, in burn treatment, 31
Skin
    benign lymphoplasias of, 20
    cancer of, 10
    inflammations that spread to, 27
Skin appendages, carcinomas of, 10
Skin biopsy, 42
Skin cancer, 10
Skin glands, rare benign tumors of, 6
Skin grafts
    in burns and scalding, 30–31
    free skin, 46
    full-thickness, 46–47
    split-thickness, 29, 47, 90–91
Skin lesions, inflammatory and functional, 25–32
Solar keratosis, 7, 10, 30, 33
Spider nevus, 21
Spiegler's tumor, 13

Spindle cell nevus, 15
Spitz tumor, 15
Split-thickness skin graft, 29, 47, 90–91
   for temporal region, 55
Squamous cell carcinoma, 3, 10, 33, 36, 41
   of lower lip, 23
Striation marks, 84
Strawberry angioma, 21
Sturge-Weber syndrome, 23
Superextension, in general anesthesia, 37
Surgical techniques, in dermatosurgery, 42–46
   elliptical excision with primary wound
      closure in, 42–43
   flaps in, 44–46
   skin biopsy in, 42
Sutton's halo nevus, 14
Suture dehiscence, 31
Sutures
   interrupted, 41
   mattress, 41
Sweat glands, inflammations originating in, 26
Syphilis, 9
Syringocystadenoma papilliferum, 6

T

Talcum granuloma, 38
Tar keratoses, 8–9
Tattoos, as foreign body intrusion, 30
Teleangiectatic nevus, 23
Temporal region, flaps for, 53–55
Testicular biopsy, 89
Thalomonal, 37
Thiersch's grafts, 29
Thin labium, correction of, 70
Thorax area, rotation flap technique for, 84
Throat, rotation flap technique for, 82
Thrombophlebitis, superficial, 28
Toenail, ingrown, 32, 92
Traumatic epithelial cysts, 30
Transposition flap technique, 46
   auricle and, 78–80
   for axilla, 85
   for cheeks, 75
   for extremities, 90–92
   for eyelids, 24, 71–72
   for hands, 92
   for lower eyelid, 72
   for lower lip defects, 67
   subcutaneous fat and, 82–83
   for trunk, 83
   for upper lip repair, 68
Trauma, lesions due to, 30
Trendelenburg flap, 62
   of auricle, 76

Triangular excision
   for auricle and related areas, 75
   for hands or feet, 92
   for lips, 65–66
   nail extraction and, 92
Trichoepithelioma, 13
Trichofolliculoma, 6
Trichophytia, deep, 25
Trunk, flap techniques for, 83–85
Tubed pedicled flaps, 47
Tuberculosis cutis colliquativa, 27
Tuberculosis cutis luposa, 26
Tubernodus angioma, 22
Tumors, 3–24
   benign, see Benign tumors
   benign epithelial, 3–6
   glomus, 22
   of nerves and nerve sheaths, 24
   of pigment-producing cells, 14–17
   vascular, 23
Tunnel flap techniques
   for auricle, 79–81
   for nose, 61–62
Tyloma, 30
Tylositas articuli, 24

U

U-flap technique, see Advancement flap
      technique, and lateral advancement flap
      technique
Ulcer, decubital, 83
Ulcus cruris venosum, 29
Ulcus rodens, 12
Unguis incarnatus, see toenail, ingrown
Unna's blackhead expressor, 26
Unna's pale teleangiectatic nevus, 23
Upper lip repair
   see also Lip; Lower lip
   advancement flap technique for, 68–69
   transposition flap technique for, 68

V

Varicocele, surgery for, 89
Varicose dilatations, of cutaneous veins, 28–29
Varicosis, in chronic venous insufficiency, 28
Vascular nevus, 23
Venous insufficiency, varicosis in, 28
Vermilionectomy, for lower lip, 64–65
Verruca filiformis, 4
Verruca plana, 4
Verruca seborrheica, 3–4
Verruca vulgaris, 3–4
Verrucous epidermal nevus, 5

Virus papilloma, 4
Virus warts, 4
Vulvectomy, 90
VY-flap technique, 44
    for hands and feet, 92

W
Wart(s)
  fig, 5
  plantar, 5
  treatment of, 4
  water, 5
Wart tinctures, 4

Water wart, 5
Wolfe-Krause full-thickness grafts, 90–91
Wounds, treatment for, 31
Wrinkles, 32

X
Xanthelasmas, 18
Xantomas, 18
X-ray therapy, avoidance of, 15

Z
Z-flap technique, 44

Plates

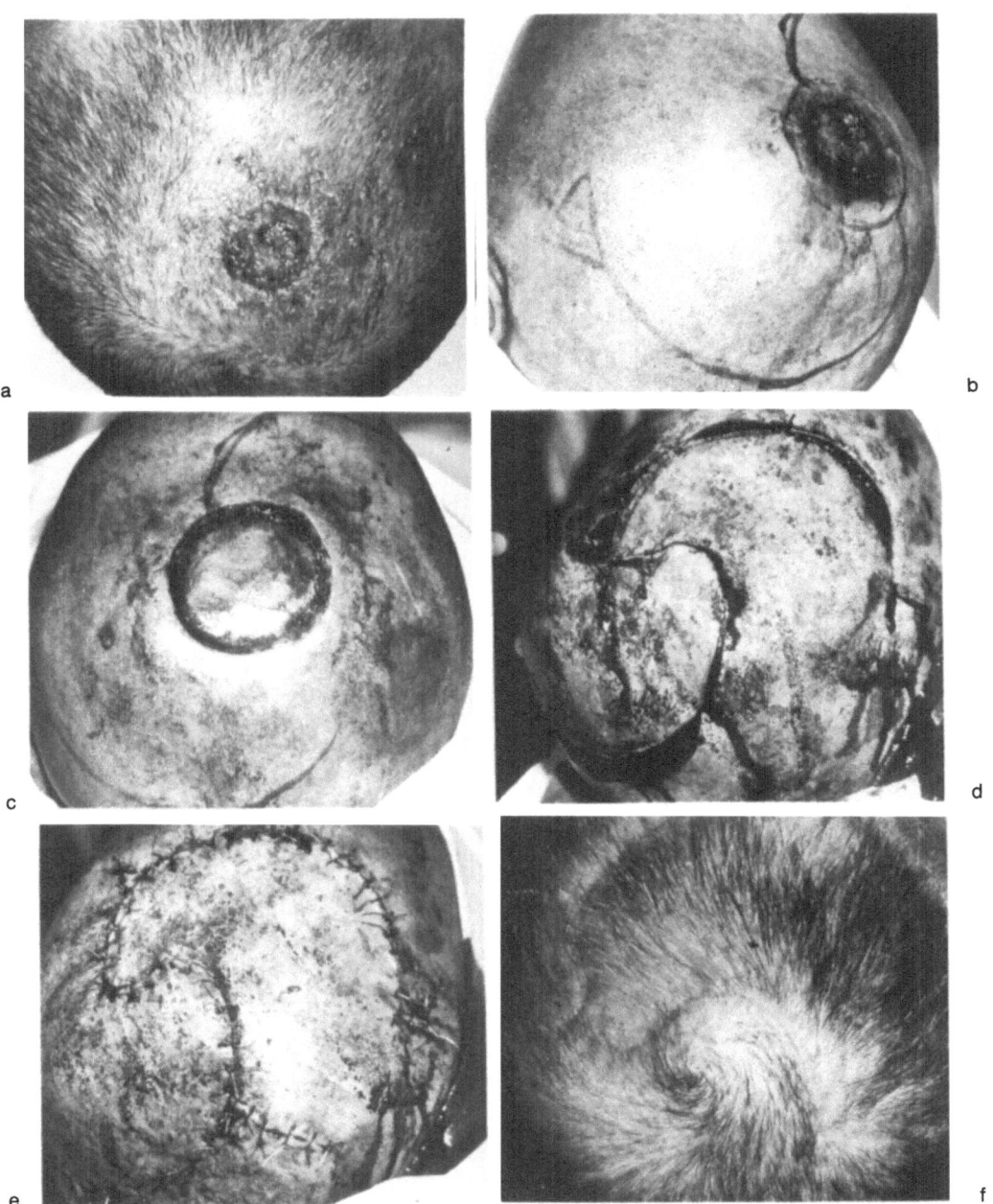

Plate 1. (cf. p. 51) L.E., 58-year-old man. Basal cell carcinoma in the scalp area: *a*, preoperative condition; *b*, planning the operation; *c*, operation defect; *d*, condition after the placing of two rotation flaps in the operation defect; *e*, condition after the covering of the operation defect by means of frontal and occipital double rotation flaps; *f*, condition 2 months postoperatively.

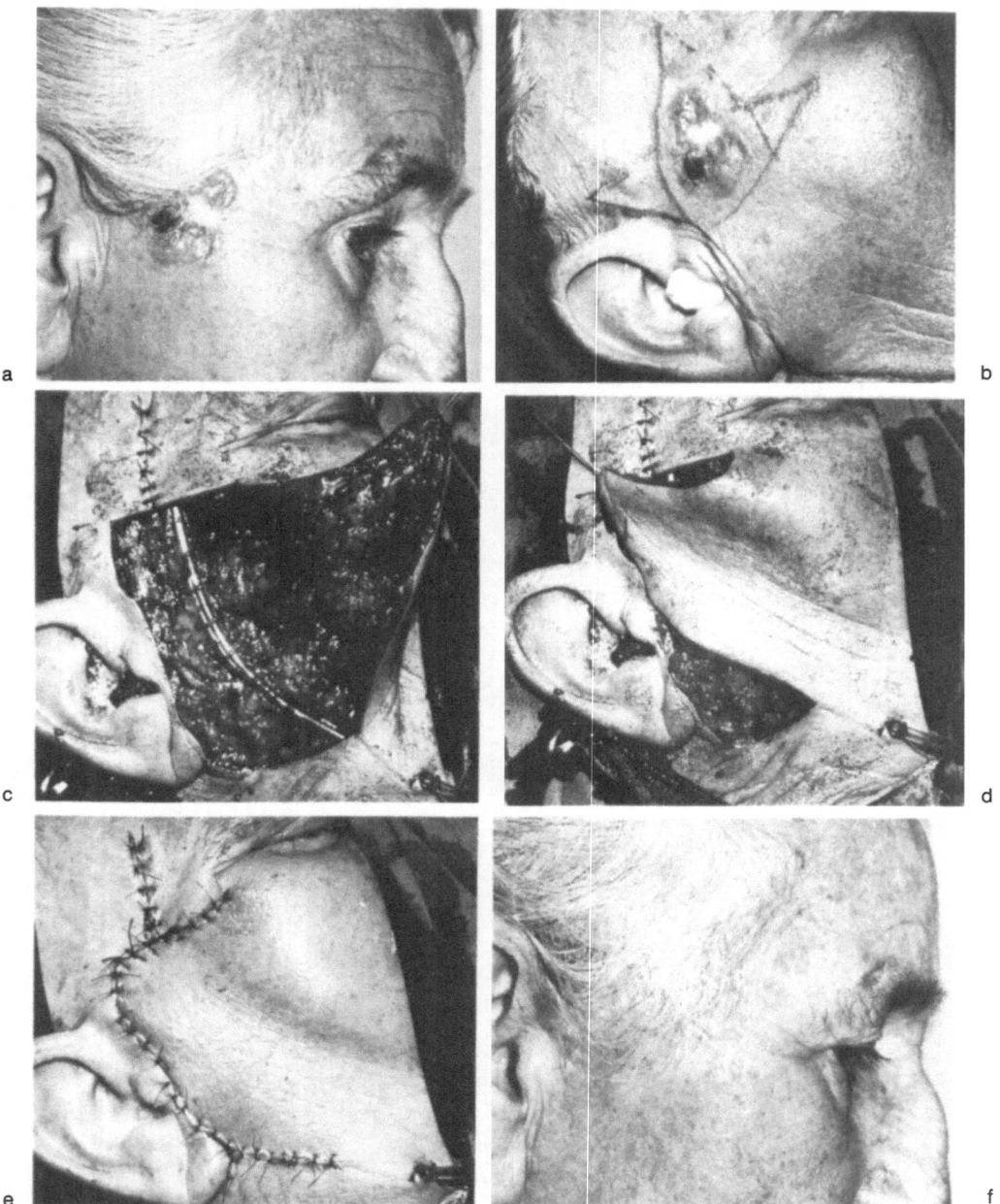

Plate 2. (cf. p. 53) L.I., 60-year-old woman. Basal cell carcinoma, right temple. *a*, preoperative condition; *b*, planning the operation; the preauricular defect is covered by means of a caudal transposition flap and the temporal defect by a dorsal transposition flap; *c*, the closed temporal defect; the caudal transposition flap prepared; *d*, the caudal transposition flap brought into position; *e*, postoperative condition after the subauricular application of a Burow's triangle; *f*, final condition 1 year postoperatively.

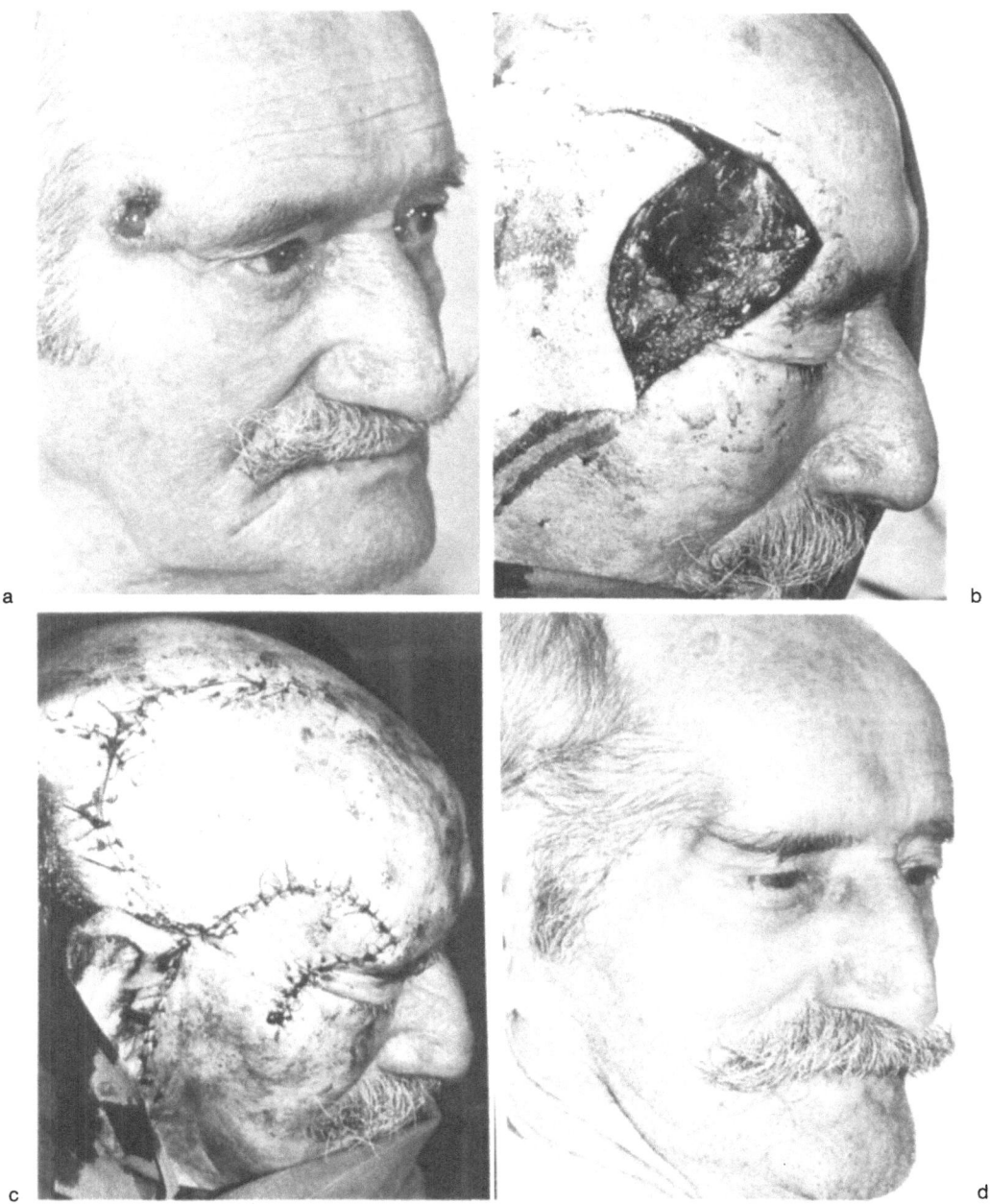

Plate 3. (cf. p. 55) D.O., 82-year-old man. Basal cell carcinoma, right temple: *a*, preoperative condition; *2*, findings following triangular excision of the focus; *c*, condition following repair of the operation defect by combined caudal and frontoparietal advancement-rotation flap; *d*, condition 12 months postoperatively.

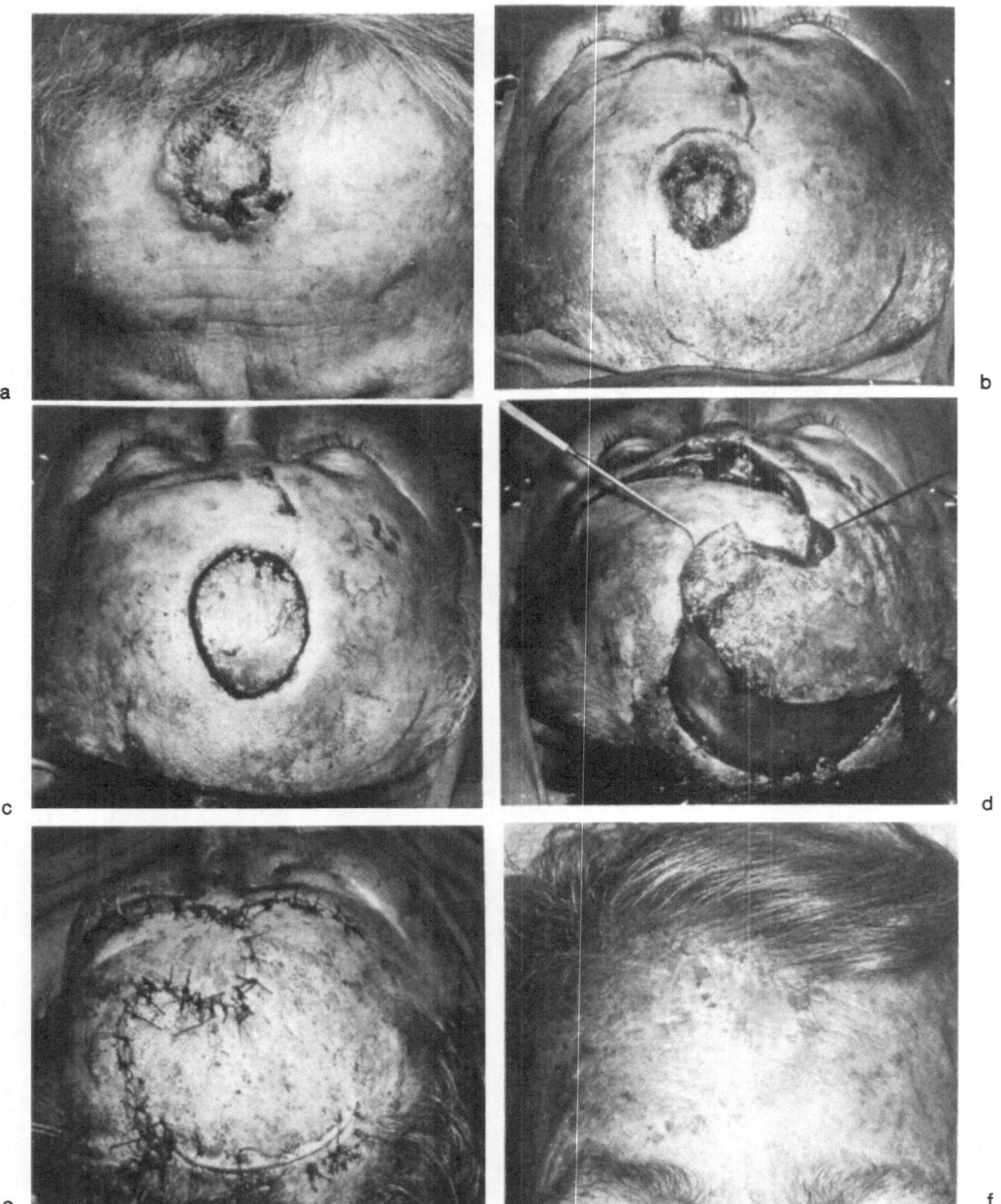

Plate 4. (cf. p. 56) W.N., 71-year-old woman. Keratoacanthoma of the middle forehead: *a*, preoperative condition; *b*, planning of the operation—double transposition flaps; *c*, operation defect; *d*, transposition from opposite directions of the two flaps of skin; *e*, condition after the covering of the operation defect; *f*, final condition 3 years postoperatively.

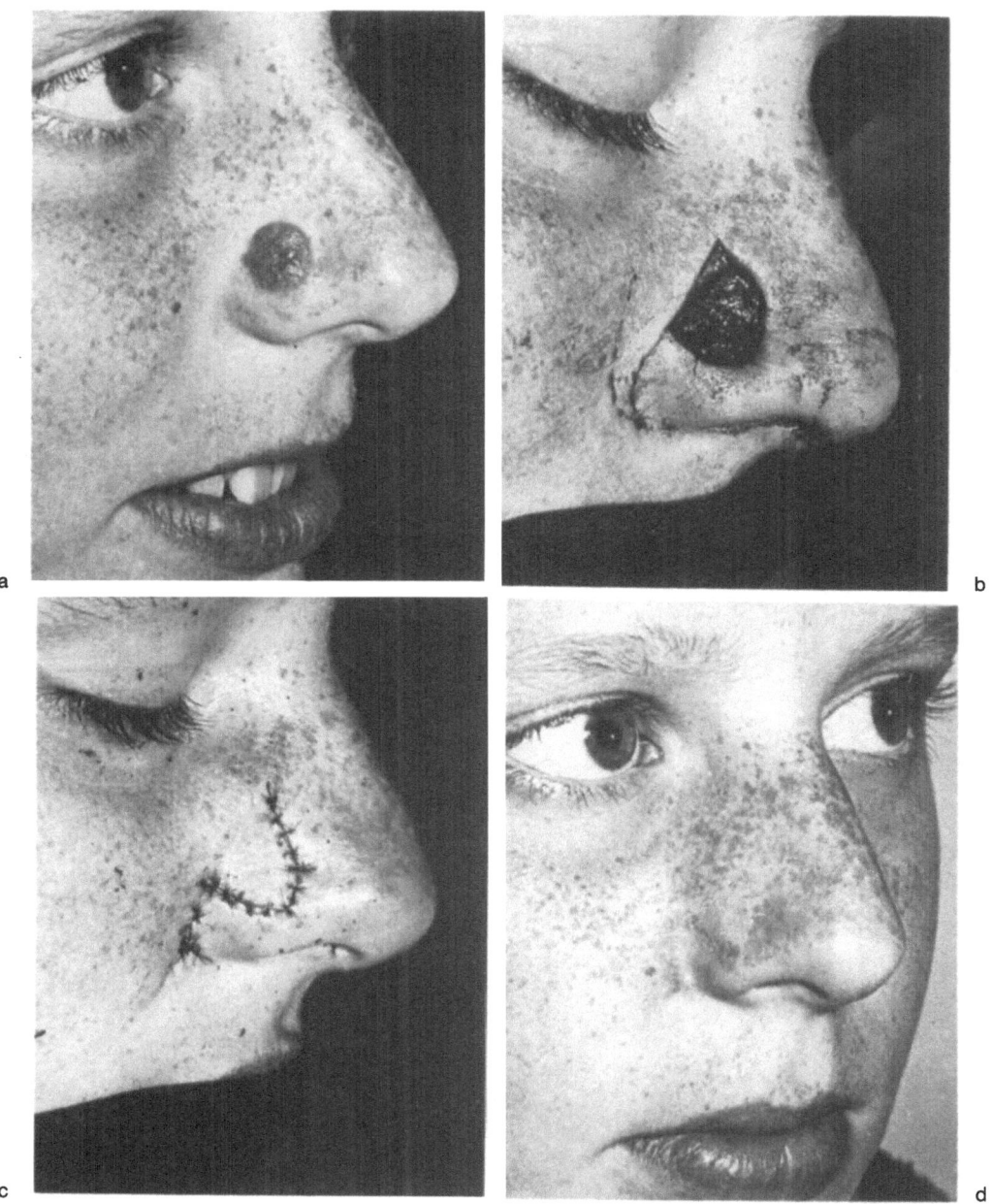

Plate 5. (cf. p. 57) Sch.D., 11-year-old boy. Juvenile melanoma of the right ala nasi; *a,* preoperative condition; *b,* condition after the excision of the focus and the preparation of a nasolabial transposition flap; *c,* condition at the end of the operation; *d,* condition 8 months postoperatively.

125

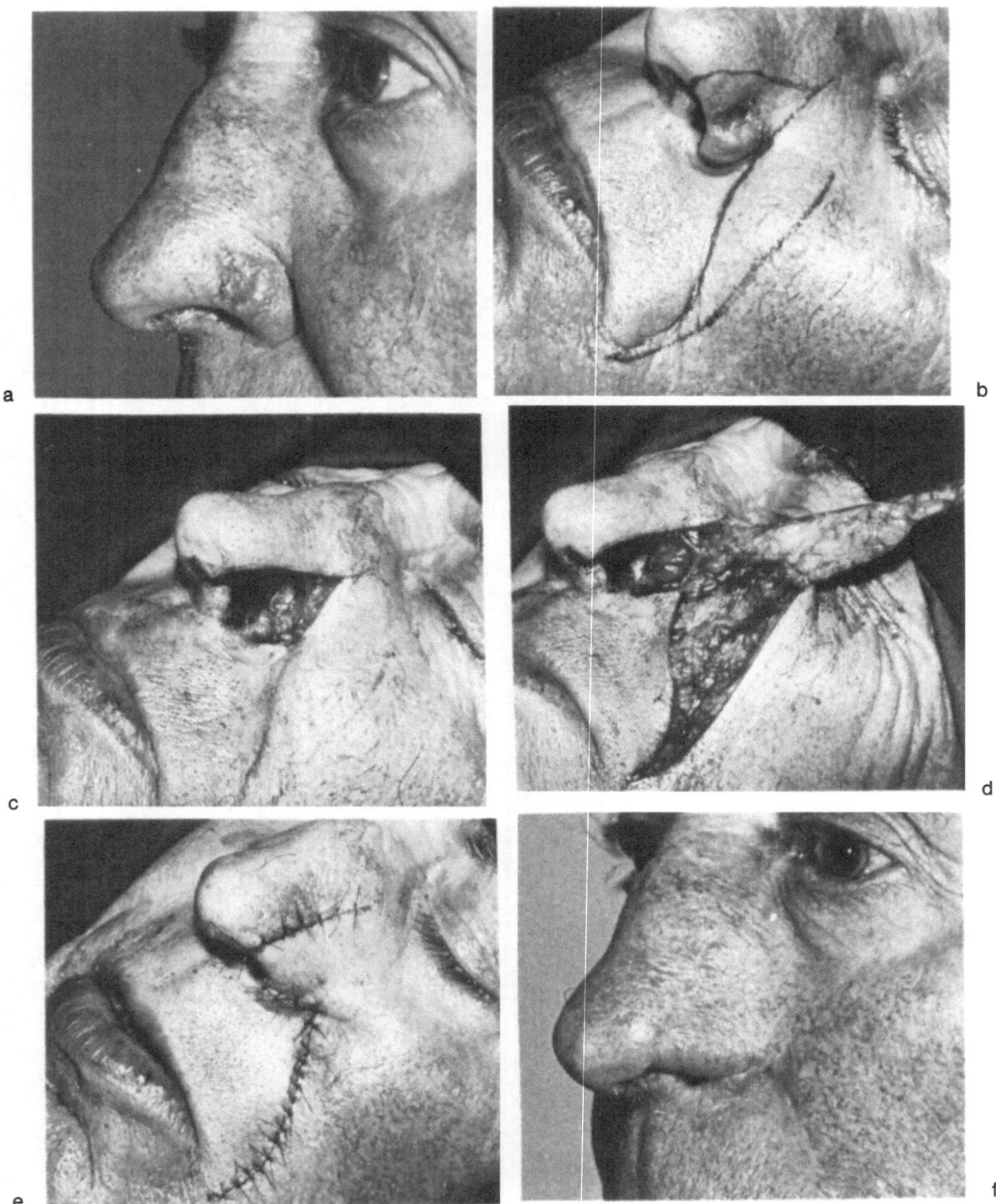

Plate 6. (cf. p. 58) H.G., 62-year-old man. Penetrating basal cell carcinoma of the left ala nasi. *a.* Before the operation: *b,* planning the operation—transposition flap; *c,* operation defect; *d,* condition after the preparation of the nasolabial transposition flap; *e,* condition at the end of the operation, the distal half of the nasolabial flap was used for the inner lining of the nose; *f,* condition 1 year postoperatively.

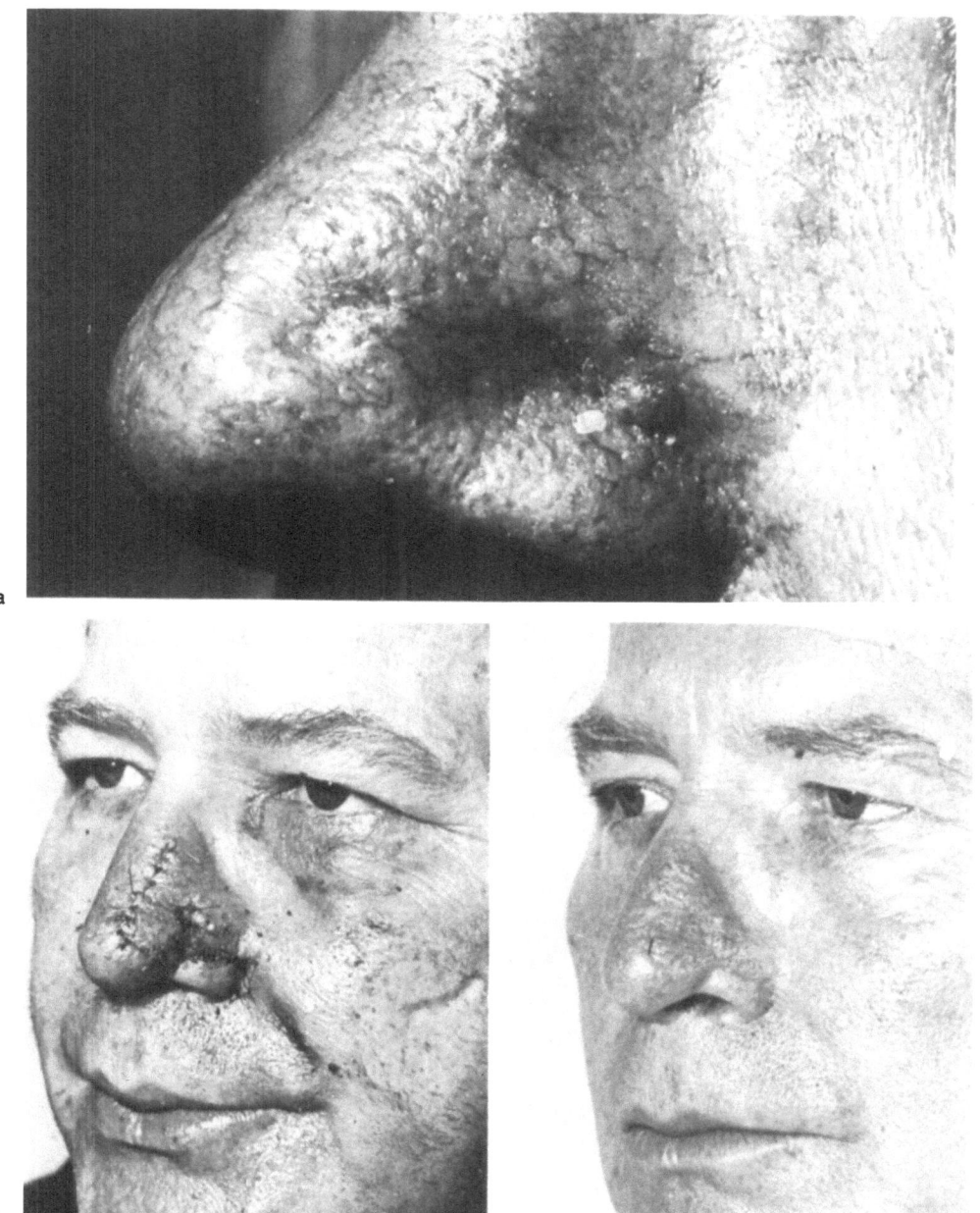

Plate 7. (cf. p. 58) F.H., 58-year-old man. Basal cell carcinoma of the left lateral tip of the nose: *a,* preoperative condition; *b,* condition 5 days following excision of the focus and repair of the defect by means of a transposition flap from the lateral nose; the secondary lateral nasal defect was treated in turn by a small transposition flap from the nasolabial region; *c,* condition 4 months postoperatively.

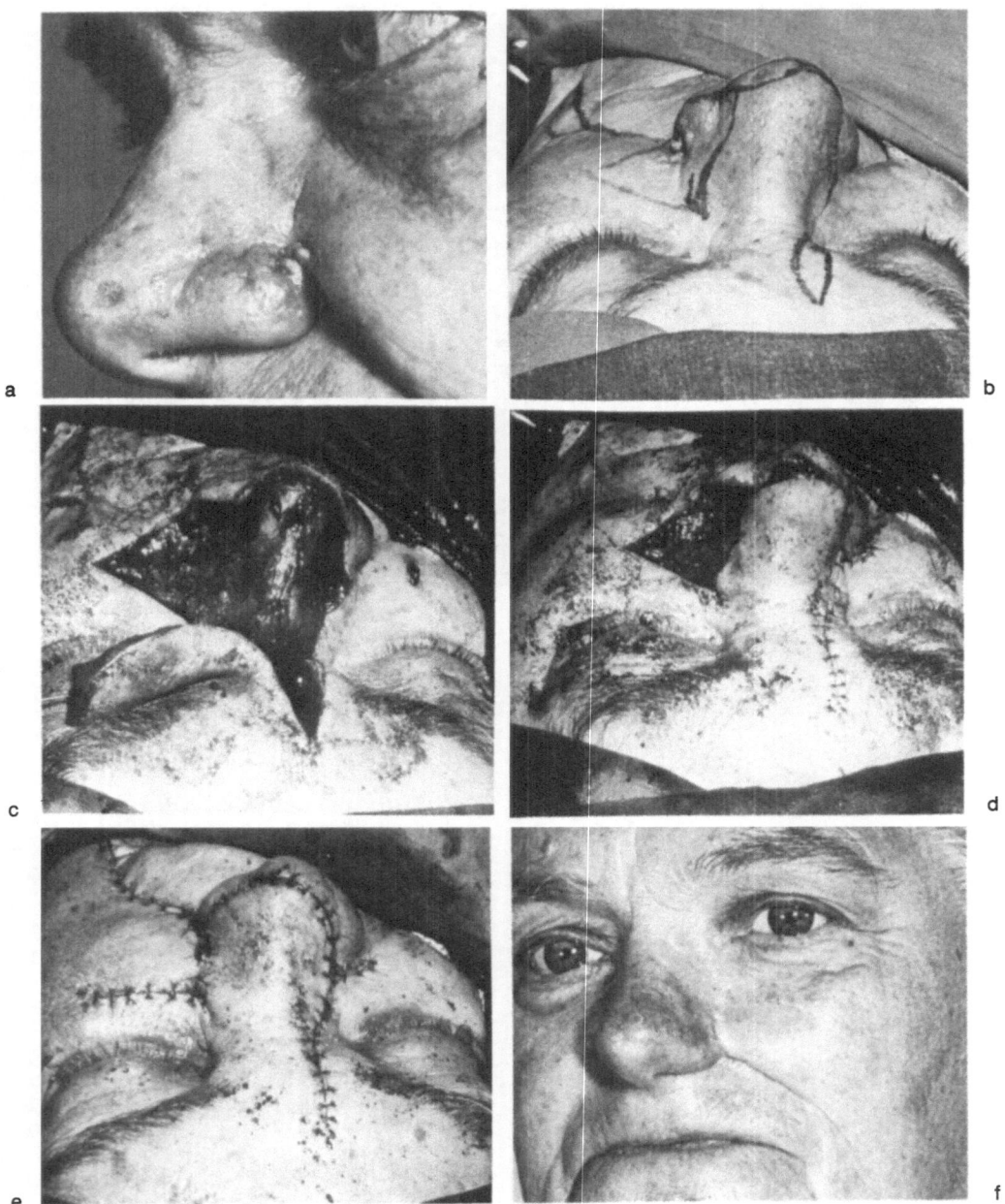

Plate 8. (cf. p. 61) G.E., 68-year-old woman. Basal cell carcinoma of the left ala nasi spreading on to the cheek: *a,* preoperative condition; *b,* planning the operation—a combination of rotation flaps from the forehead and a caudal transposition flap; *c,* operation defect with the prepared rotation flaps; *d,* rotation flaps in position; *e,* condition at the end of the operation after the covering of the remaining defect on the cheek with a caudal transposition flap; *f,* final condition 3 years postoperatively.

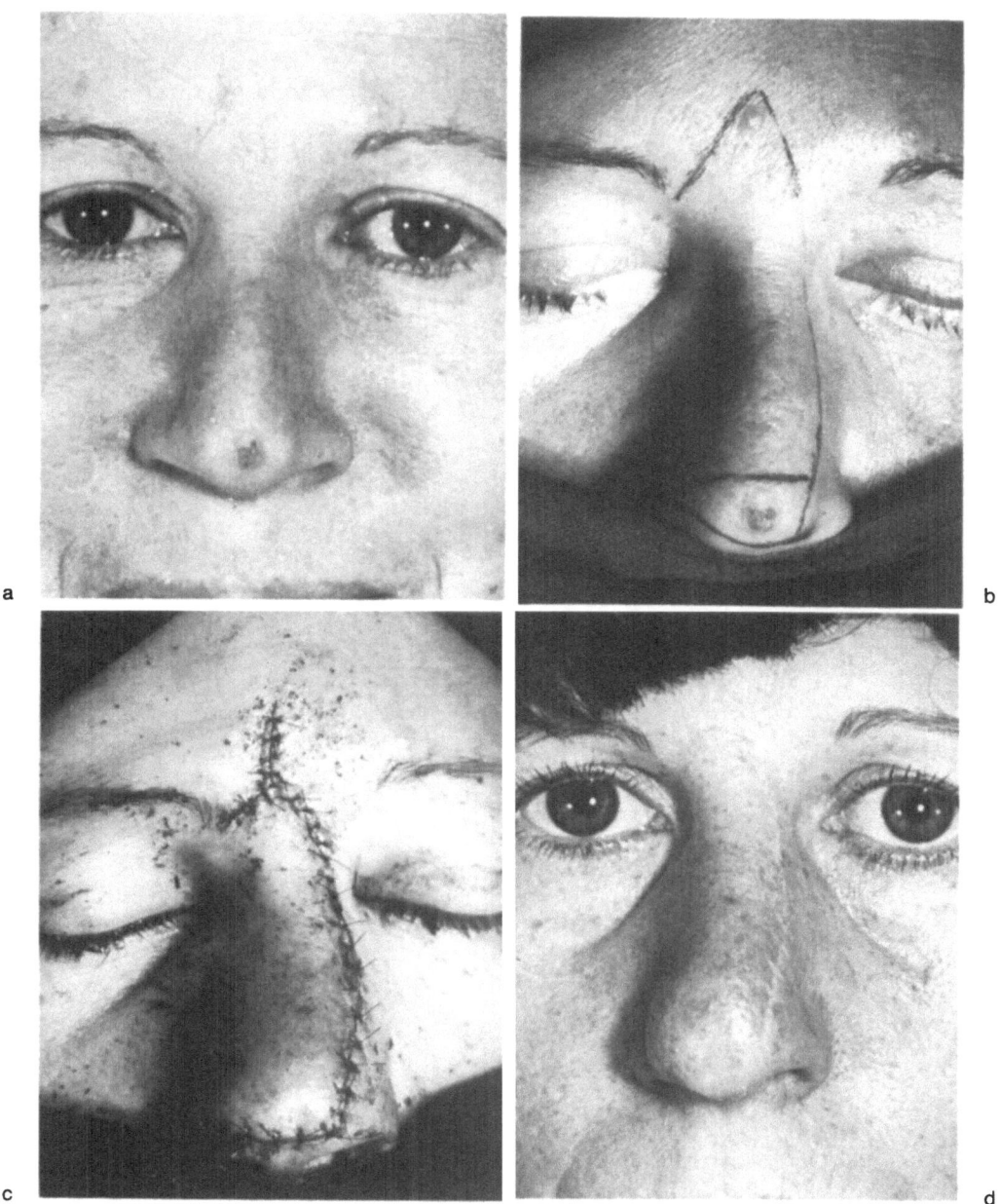

Plate 9. (cf. p. 61) H.L., 37-year-old woman. Basal cell carcinoma scarring of the tip of the nose: *a*, preoperative condition; *b*, planning the operation—rotation flap combined with a V-Y flap in the area of the glabella; *c*, condition at the end of the operation; *d*, condition 20 months post-operatively.

129

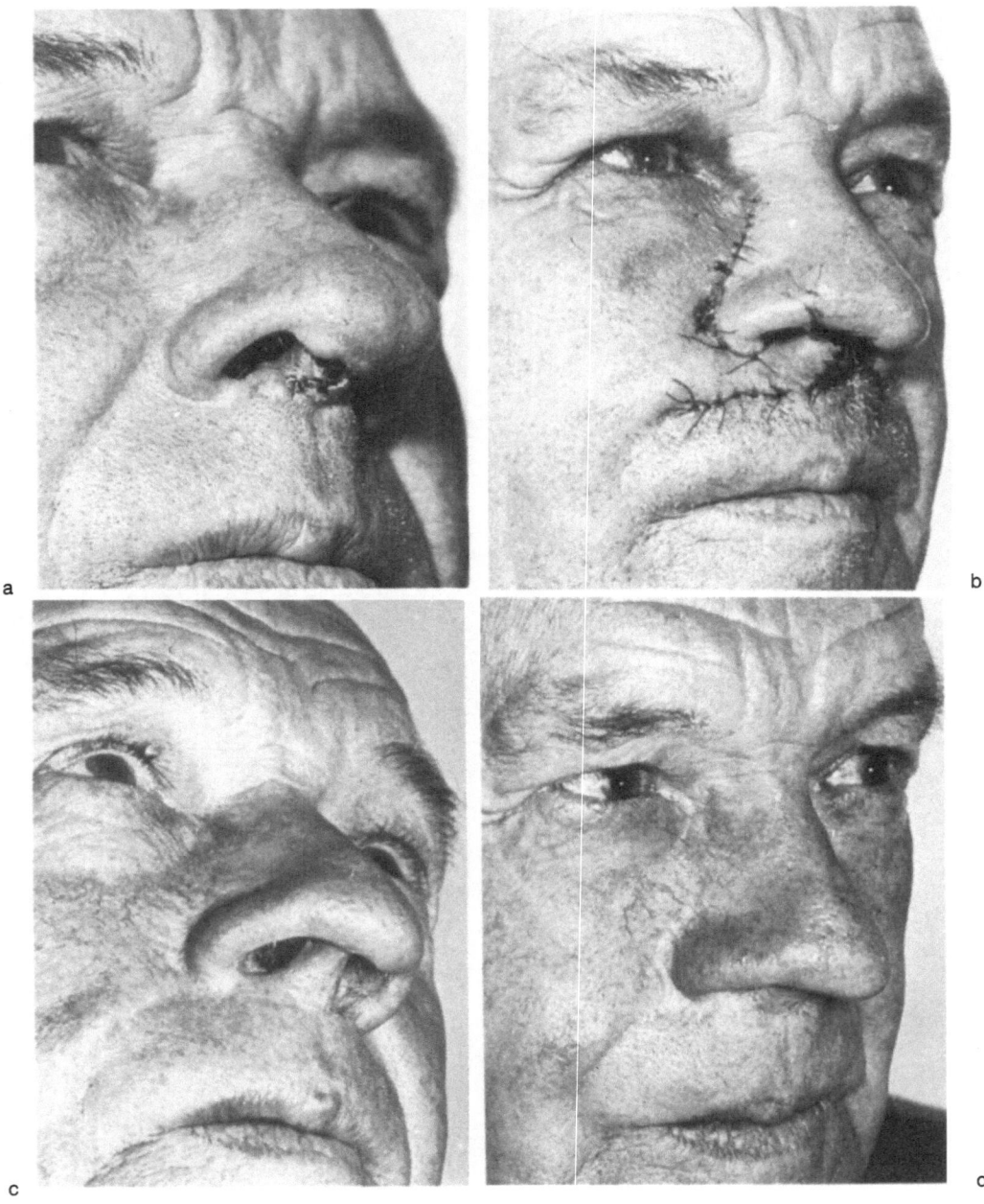

Plate 10. (cf. p. 61) K.A., 60-year-old man. Relapsed basal cell carcinoma in the area of the floor of the nose and the bridge of the nose after X-ray therapy: *a*, preoperative condition; *b*, condition after the excision of the tumor and the covering of the operation defect by means of cranial partial tunnel flaps; *c*, condition after a corrective operation to restore the nasolabialial sulcus; *d*, final condition 5 years postoperatively.

130

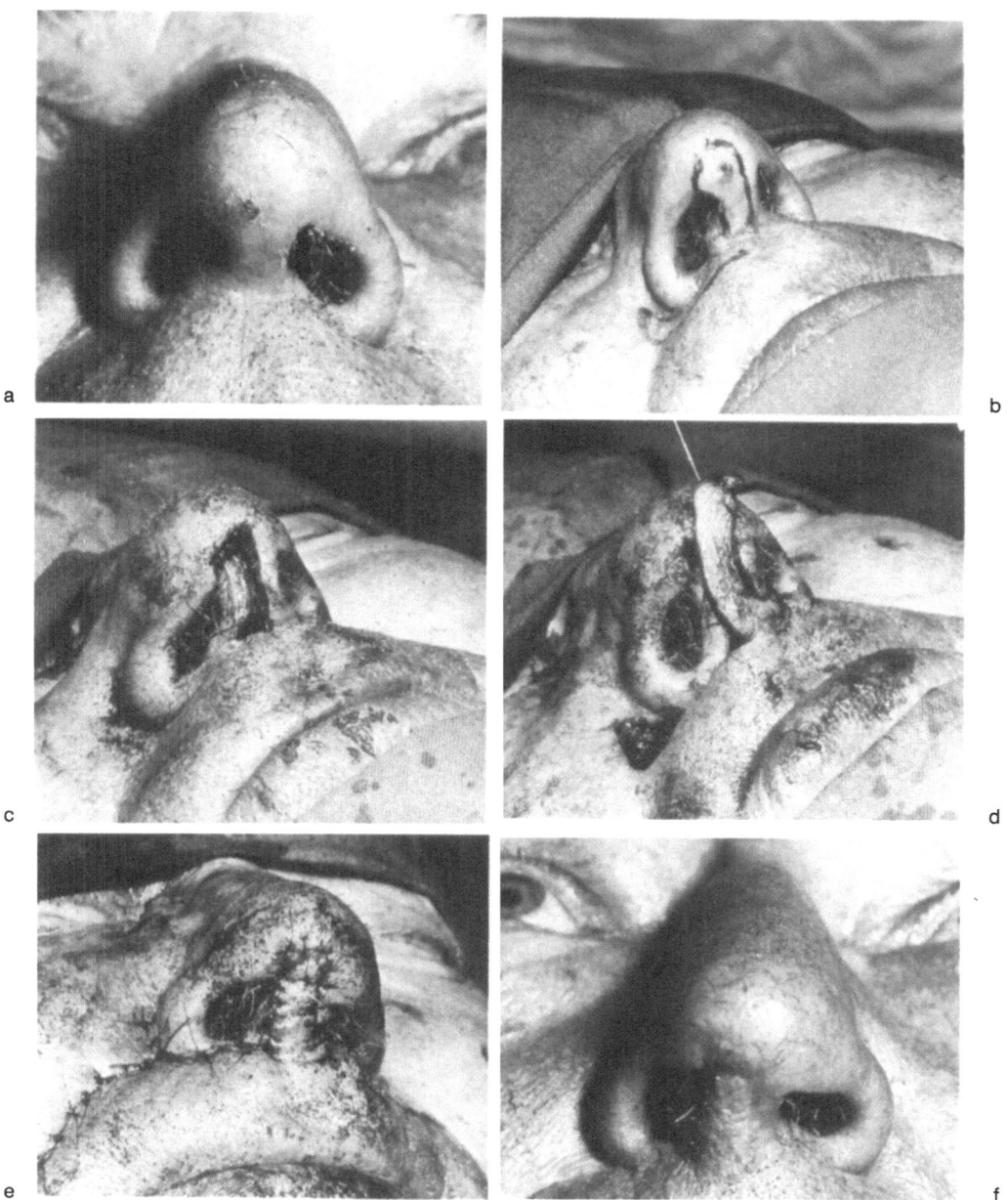

Plate 11. (cf. p. 62) T.F., 67-year-old man. Basal cell carcinoma of the bridge of the nose: *a,* preoperative condition; *b,* planning the operation—transposition flap graft from the upper lip; *c,* operation defect; *d,* transposition graft in position; *e,* condition at the end of the operation; *f,* condition 3 years postoperatively.

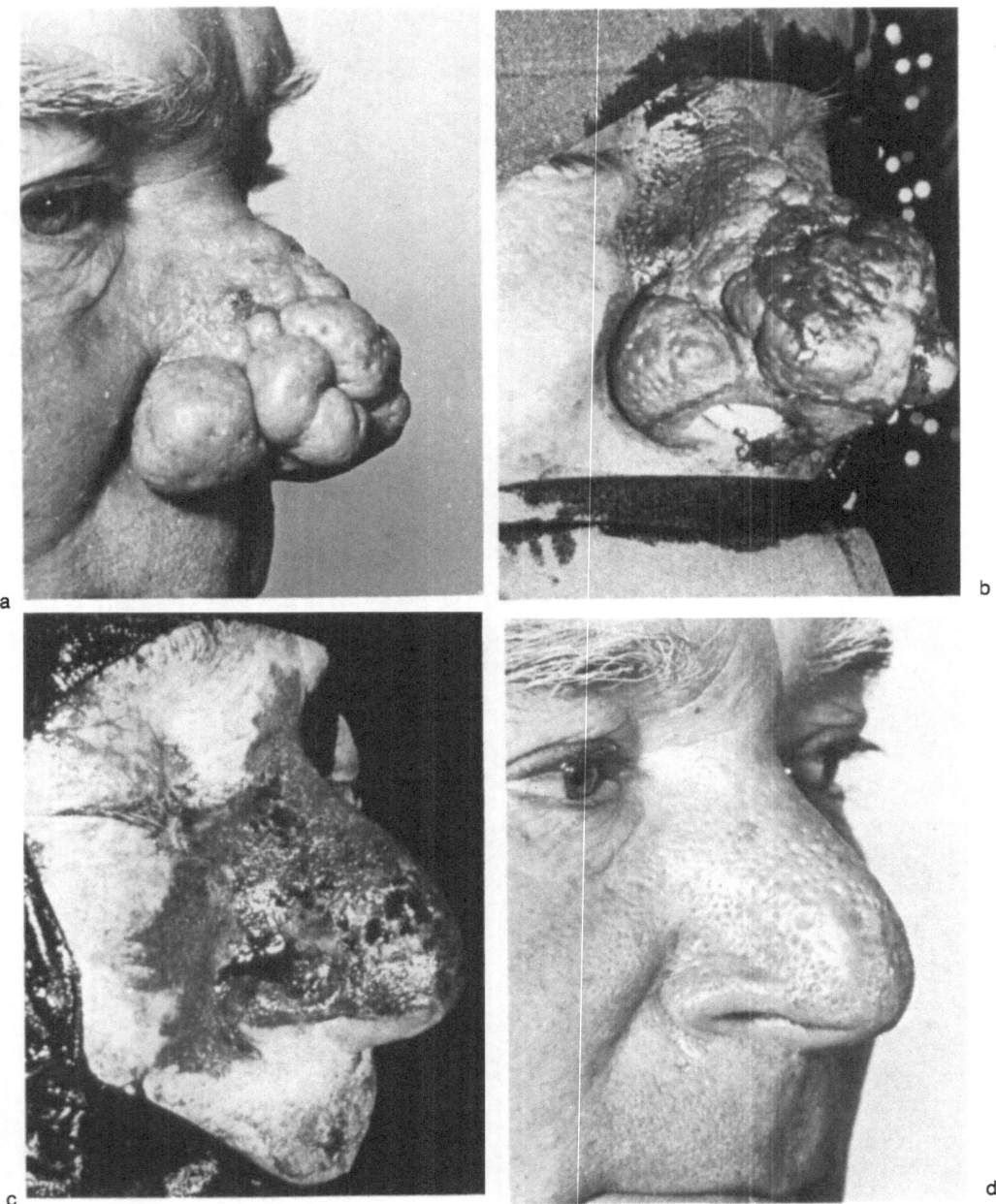

Plate 12. (cf. p. 63) K.O., 72-year-old man. Rhinophyma: *a* and *b*, preoperative condition; *c*, findings following excision of the nodules with scalpel and reshaping by means of high-speed dermabrasion; *d*, condition 6 months postoperatively.

132

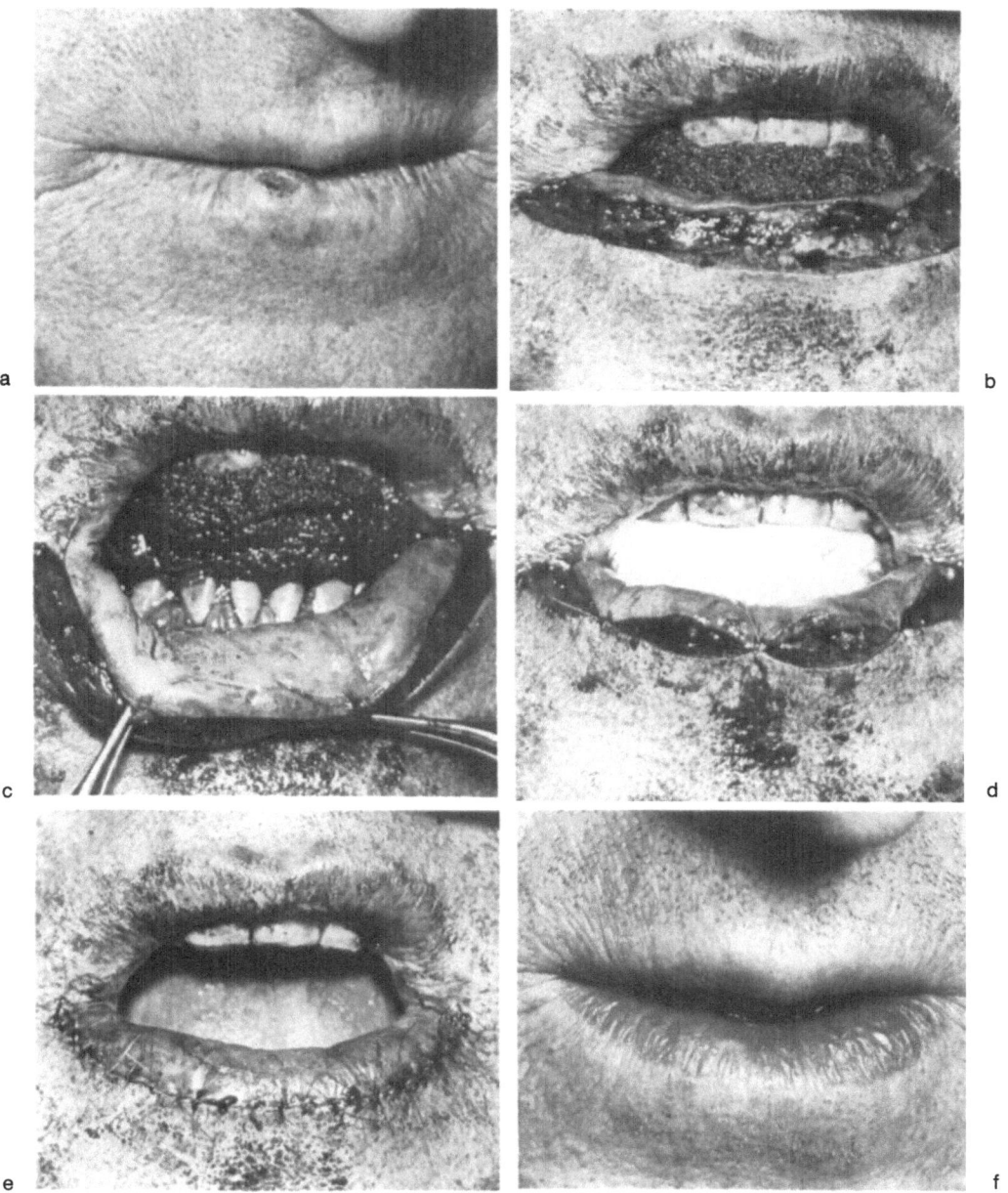

Plate 13. (cf. p. 65) D.H., 42-year-old man. Squamous cell carcinoma of the lower lip: *a*, preoperative condition; *b*, after excision of the focus, including the entire lower prolabium, according to the Langenbeck-von Bruns technique; *c*, drawing forward of the submucously mobilized buccal mucous membrane of the lower lip; *d*, affixing the mucous membrane of the lower lip with atraumatic sutures at the border of the prolabium; *e*, condition after completion of the Langenbeck-von Bruns surgical technique; *f*, condition 12 months postoperatively.

133

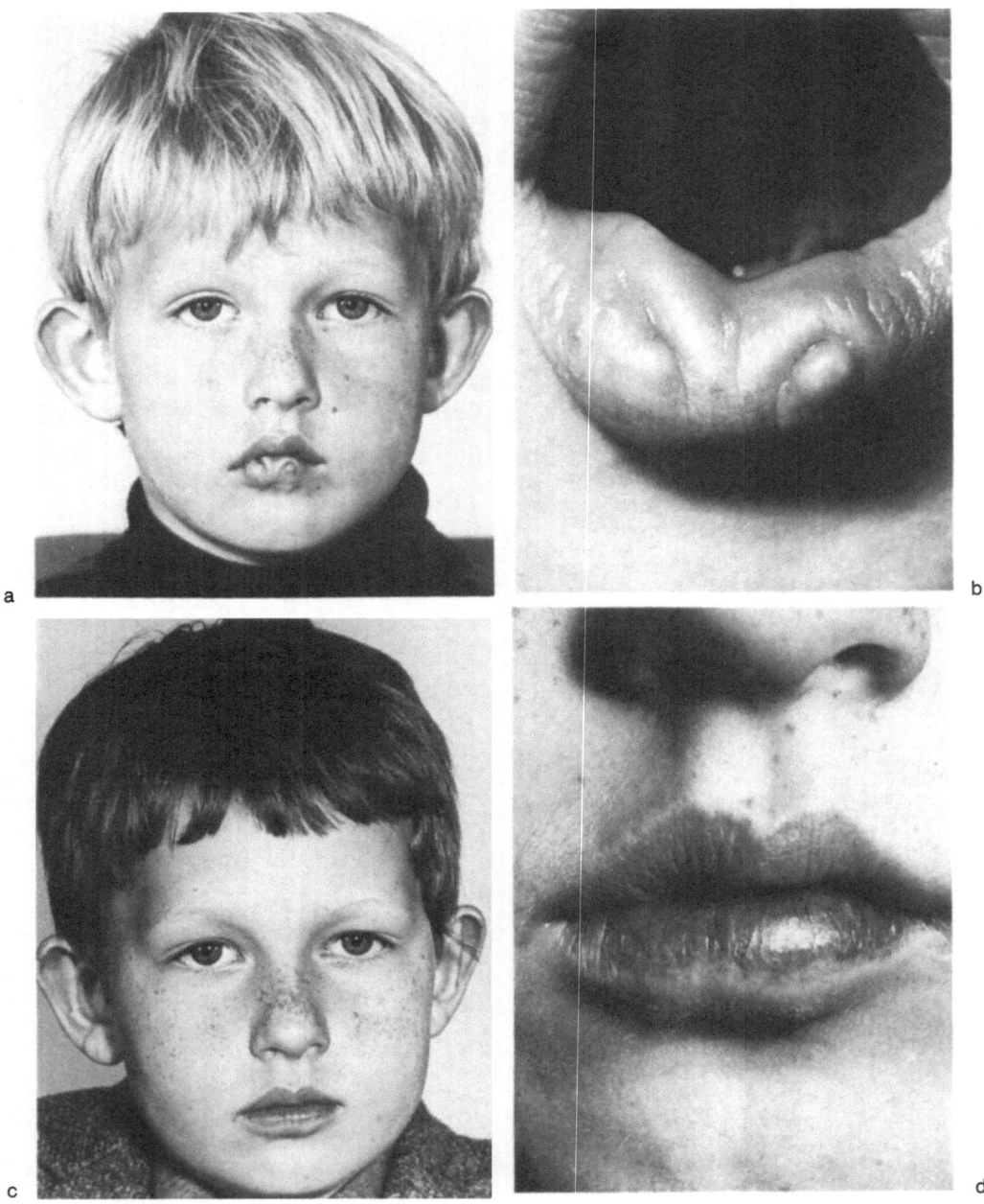

Plate 14. (cf. p. 65) A.D., 5-year-old boy. Congenital dimple of the lip: *a* and *b*, preoperative condition; *c* and *d*, condition 5 months after excision of the deformity of the lower lip and repair of the operation defect in terms of a vermillionectomy according to Langenbeck-von Bruns.

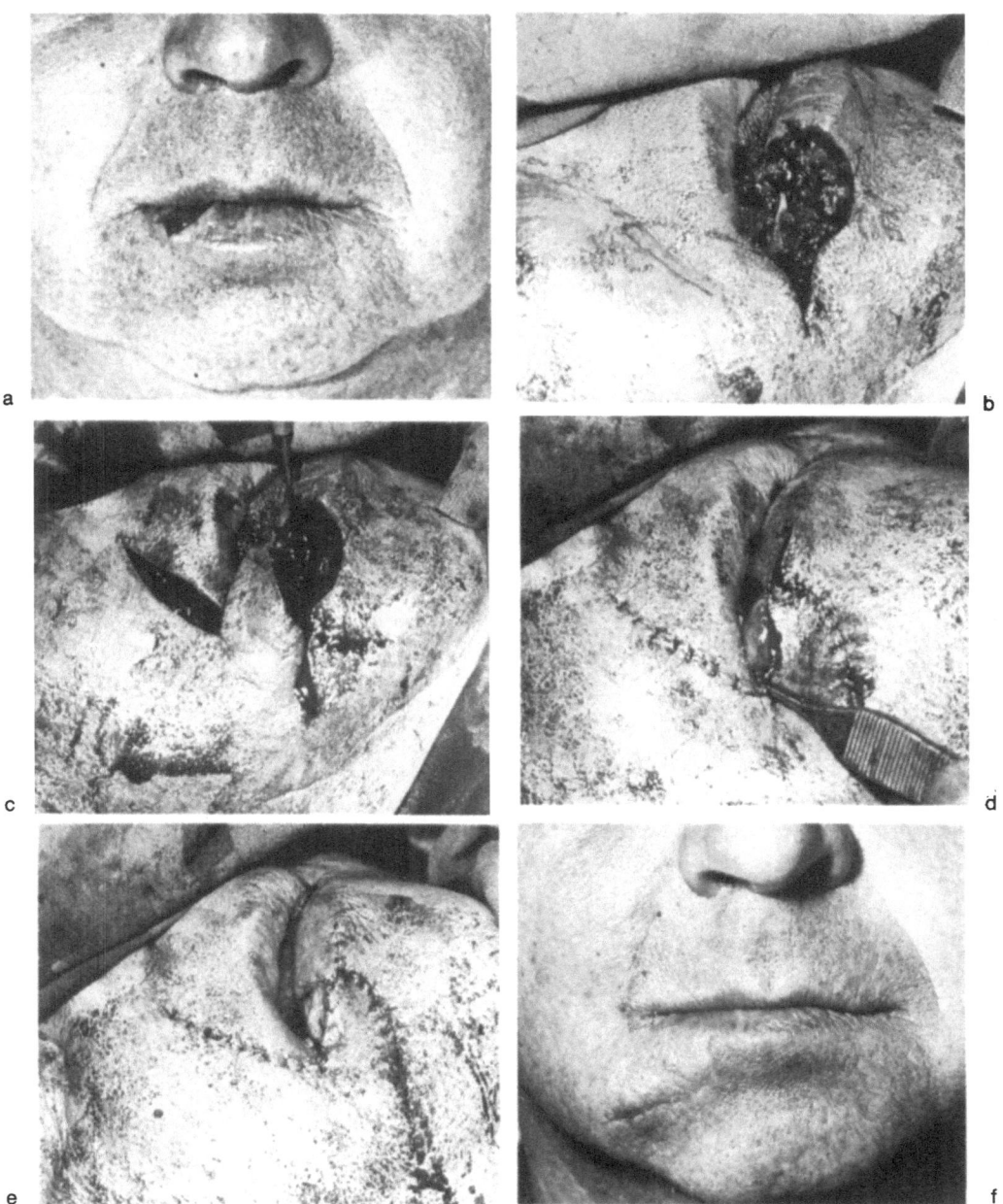

Plate 15. (cf. p. 67) K.A., 60-year-old man. Squamous cell carcinoma of the lower lip: *a*, preoperative condition; *b*, after excision of the focus; *c*, a nasolabial transposition flap is brought into the lower lip defect; *d*, reconstruction of the lower prolabium by advancement of buccal mucous membrane; *e*, condition at the end of the operation; *f*, condition 2 months postoperatively.

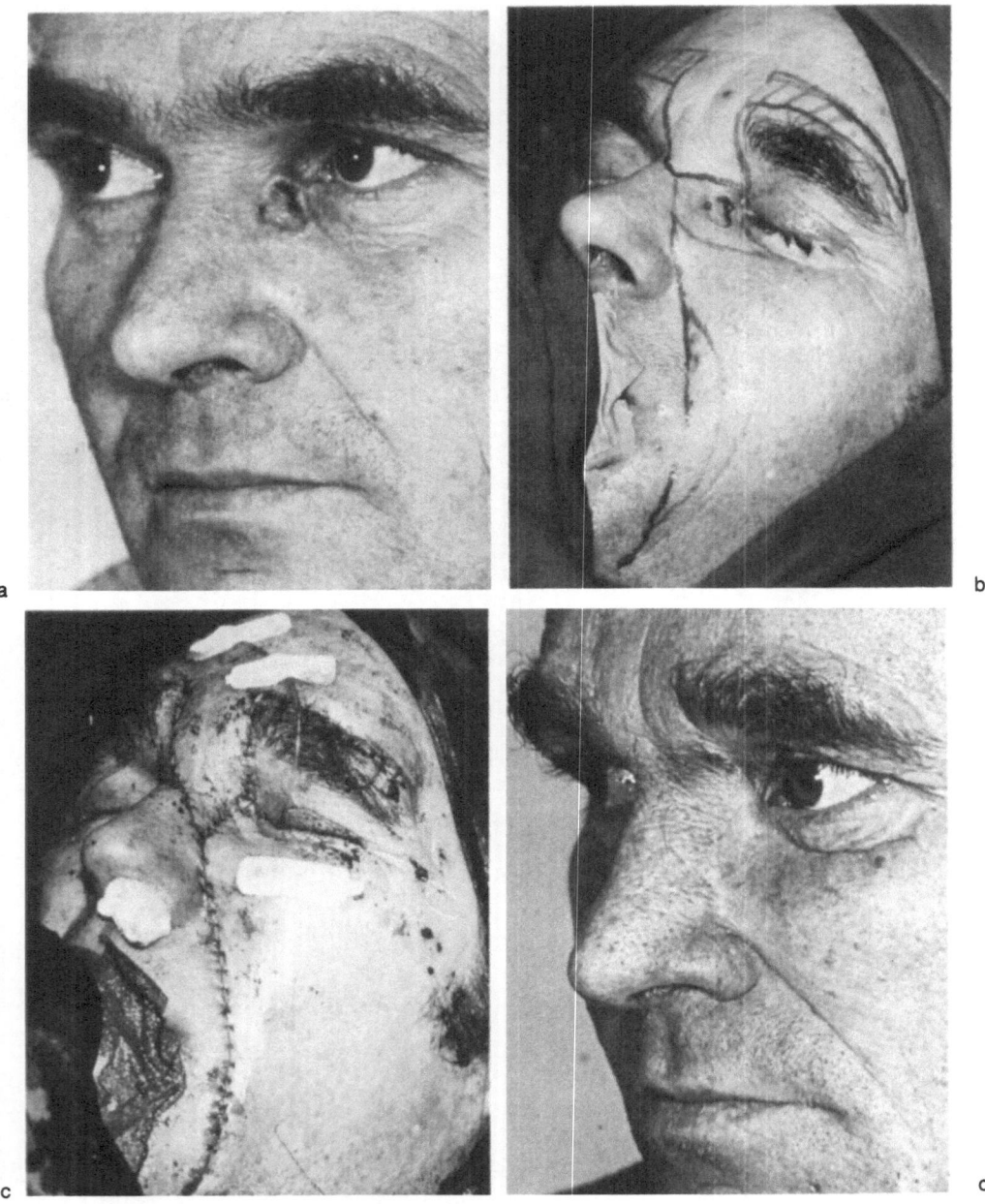

Plate 16. (cf. p. 71) H.W., 41-year-old man. Basal cell carcinoma of the medial corner of the left eyelid: *a,* preoperative condition; *b,* planning the operation—a combination of cranial and caudal transposition flaps; *c,* condition at the end of the operation, with the insertion of a silicone catheter into the tear duct; the catheter was left in situ for 2 months; *d,* final condition 2 years postoperatively.

136

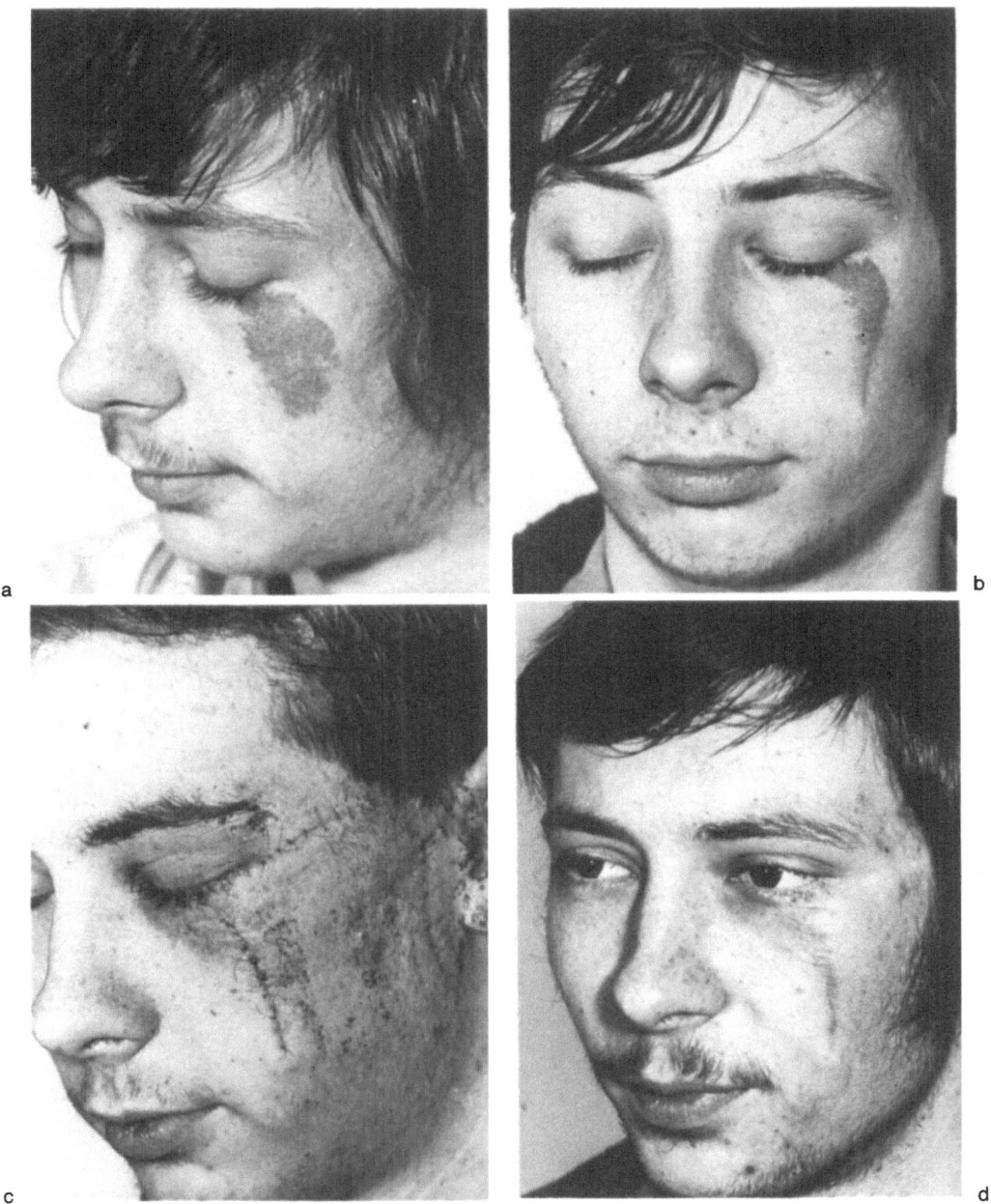

Plate 17. (cf. p. 72) F.E., 17-year-old man. Port wine stain on the left lower palpebra and the left cheek: *a*, preoperative condition; *b*, result 9 months following partial excision of the focus and repair of the defect by a Dehnungsplastik; *c*, view of the patient 4 days after excision of the remaining focus and defect repair with the aid of a rotation flap according to Imre; *d*, final condition 14 months postoperatively.

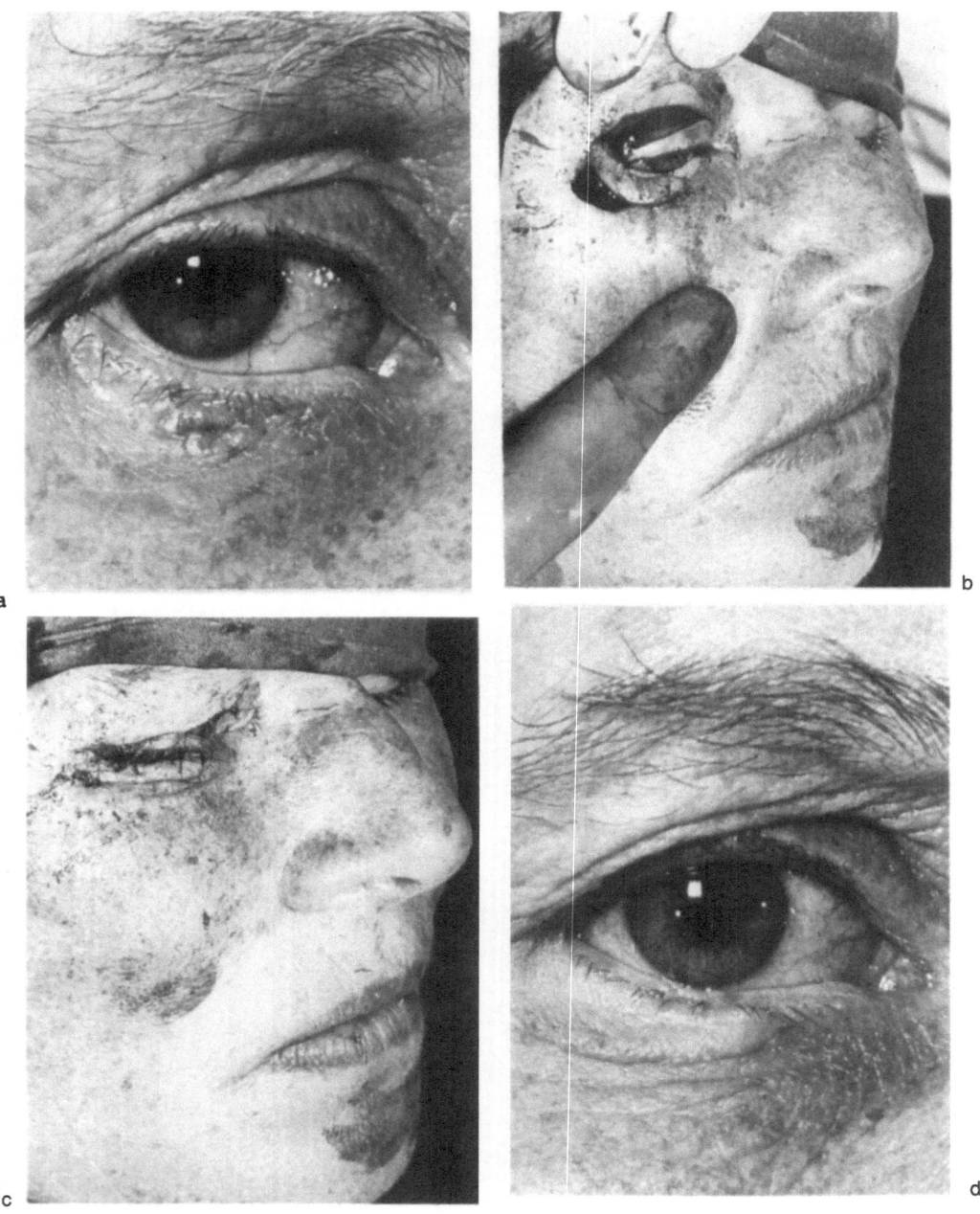

Plate 18. (cf. p. 72) E.M., 52-year-old woman. Basal cell carcinoma in the area of the right lower lid: *a,* preoperative condition, *b,* after excision of the focus and placement of a transposition flap from the upper palpebra into the lower palpebral defect; *c,* flap donor site on the upper palpebra closed by primary sutures; transposition flap affixed in the lower palpebral defect; *d,* condition 12 months postoperatively.

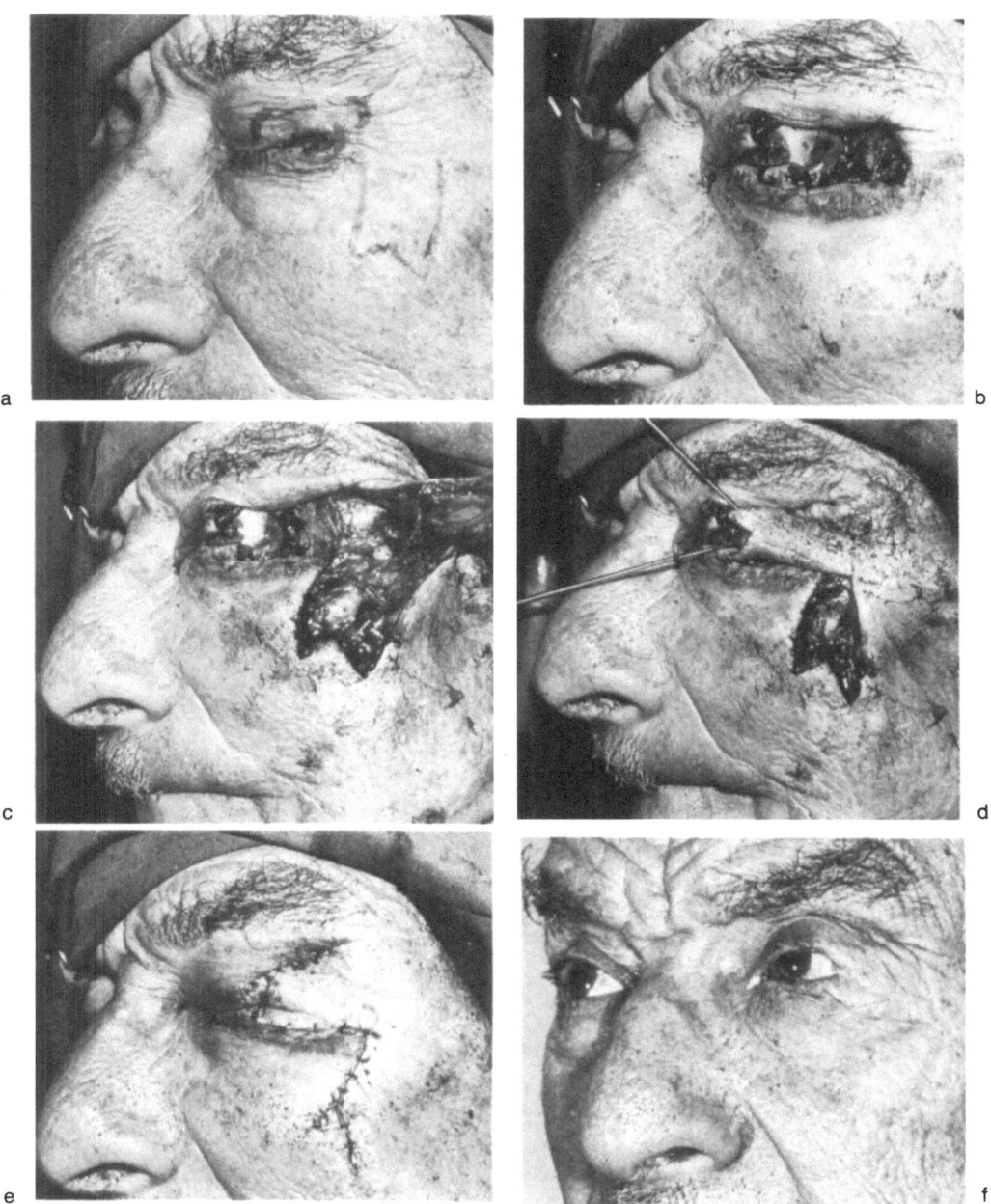

Plate 19. (cf. p. 72) M.O., 78-year-old man. Basal cell carcinoma of the outer corner of the left eyelid: *a*, preoperative condition and the planning of the operation—transposition flap from the cheek; *b*, operation defect after resection of the outer third of both the lower and the upper eyelid; *c*, transposition flap prepared; *d*, placement of the transposition flap in the operation defect; *e*, condition at the end of the operation; substitution of the conjunctiva by means of mobilization of the remaining parts; *f*, condition 18 months postoperatively.

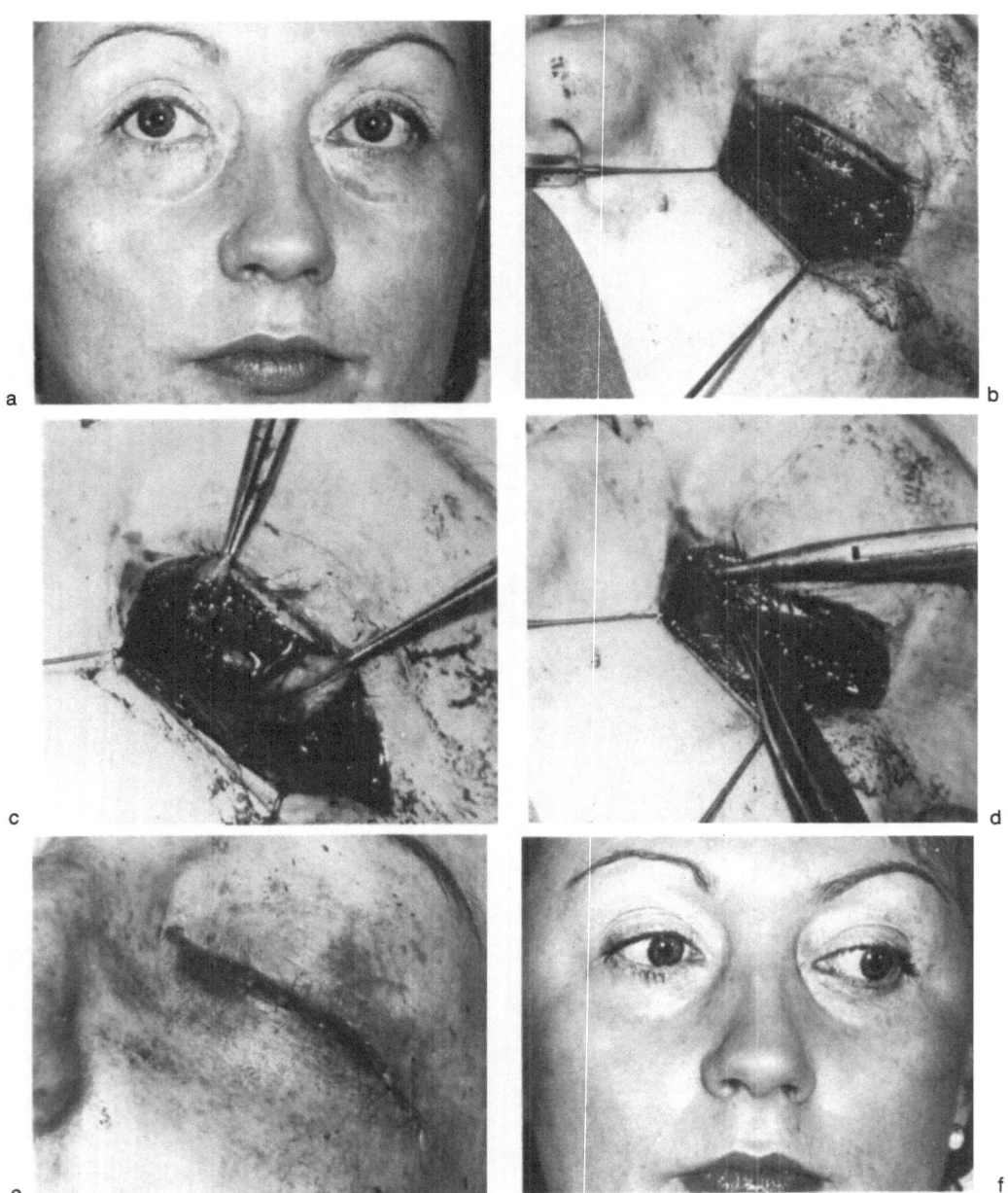

Plate 20. (cf. p. 75) G.J., 41-year-old woman. Baggy eyelids: *a,* preoperative condition; *b,* condition after mobilization of the skin of the lower eyelid; *c,* presentation of the herniated orbital fatty tissue; *d,* condition after resection of the fatty tissue and suture of the musculus orbicularis occuli; *e,* condition at the end of the operation; *f,* condition 7 months postoperatively.

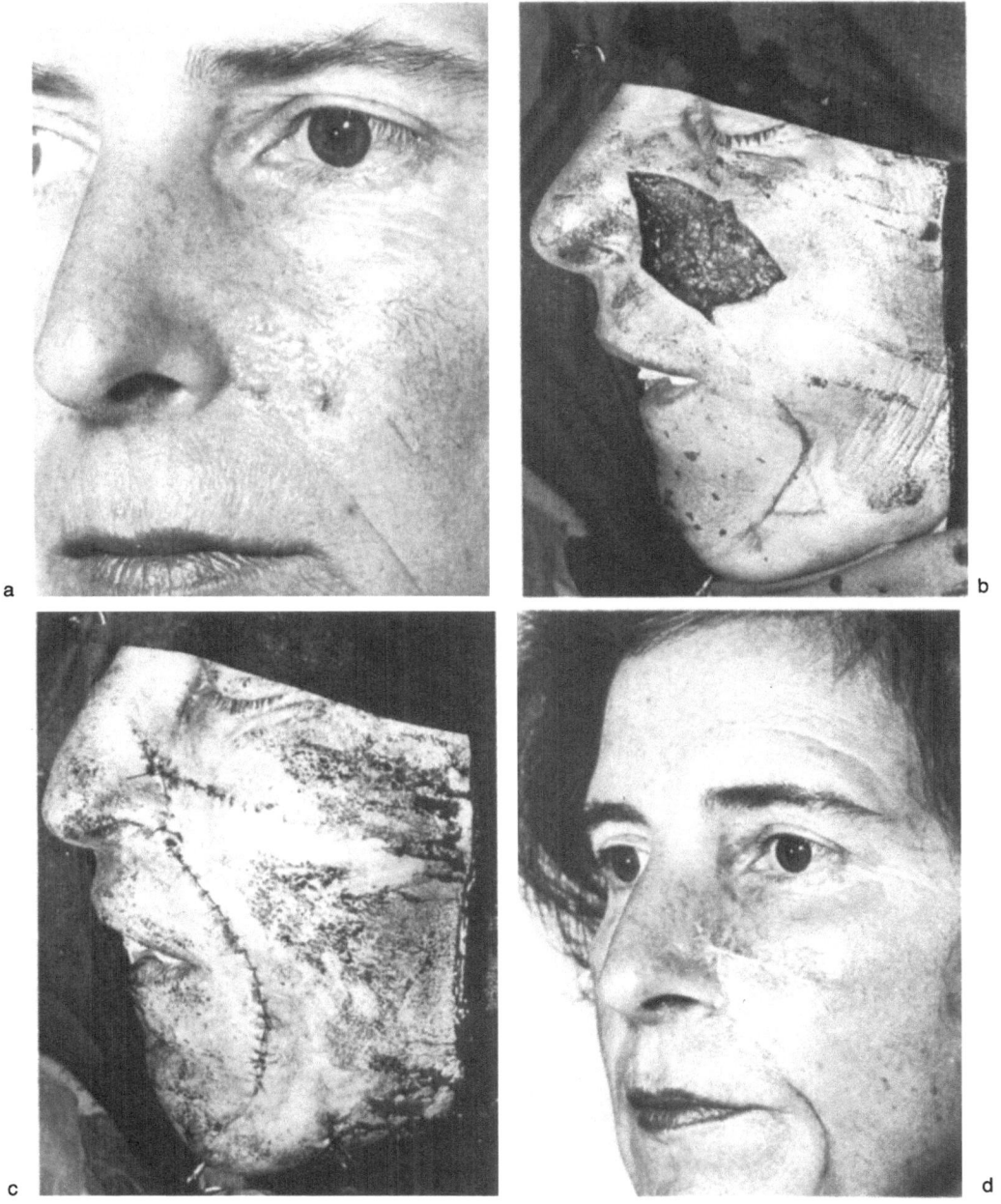

a
b
c
d

Plate 21. (cf. p. 75) D.H., 50-year-old woman. Basal cell carcinoma of the left cheek: a, preoperative condition; b, following excision of the focus; c, condition after repair of the operation defect by means of a caudal advancement flap; d, result 6 months postoperatively.

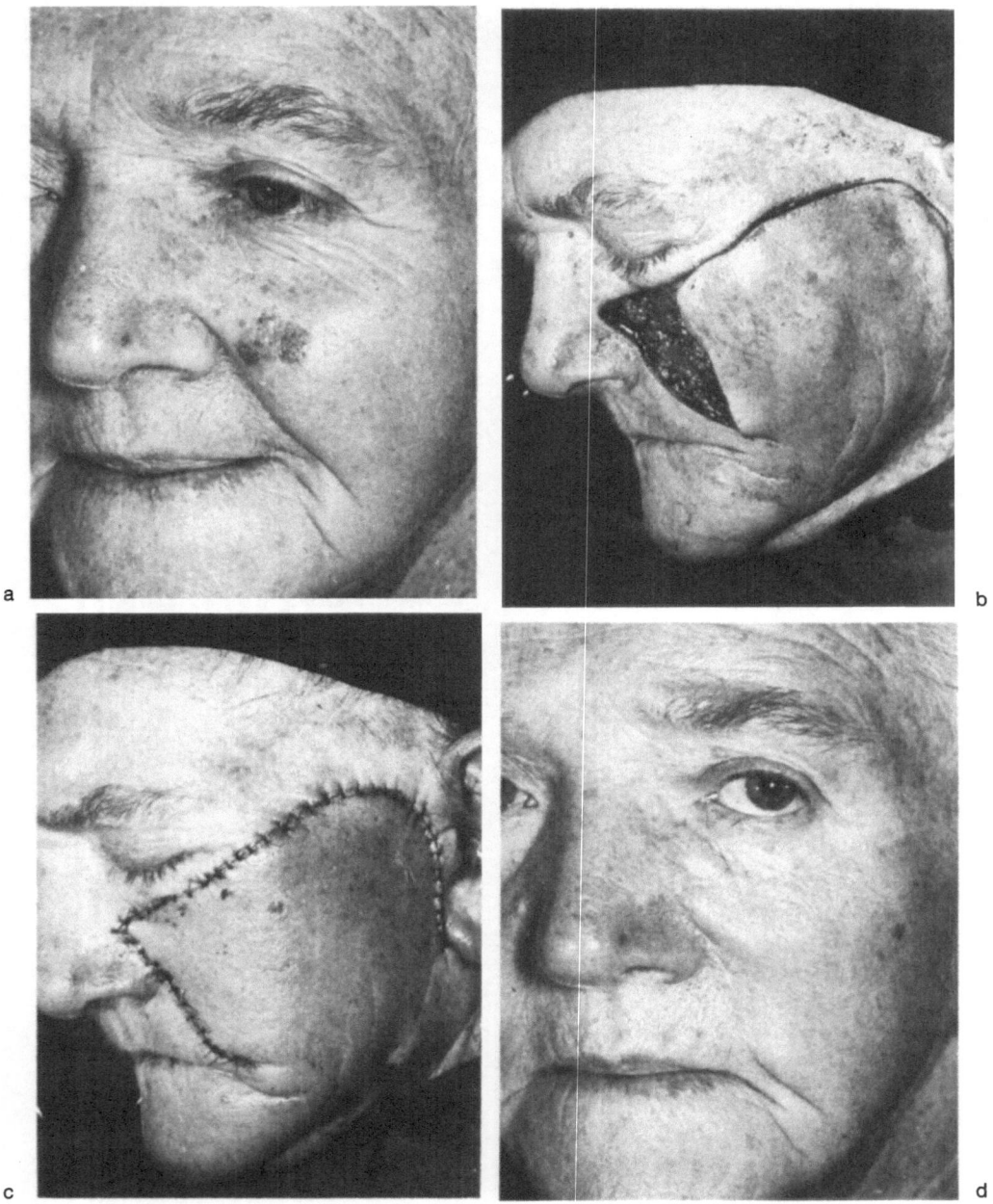

Plate 22. (cf. p. 75) W.R., 70-year-old woman. Lentigo maligna of the left cheek: *a*, preoperative condition; *b*, condition after excision of the tumor, and preparation of the cheek rotation; *c*, condition at the end of the operation after suturing the transposed rotation flap in the primary operation defect; *d*, condition 1 year postoperatively.

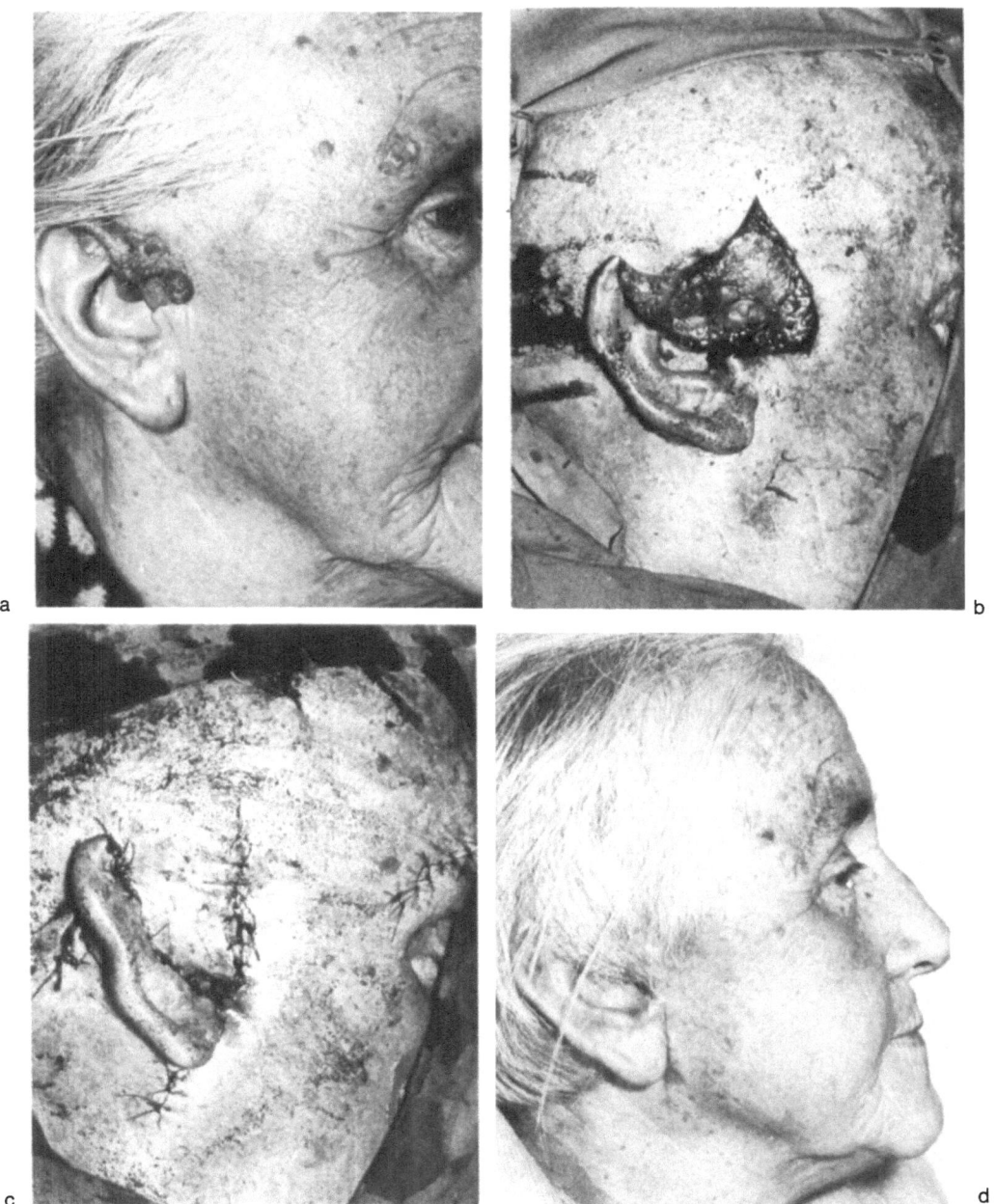

Plate 23. (cf. p. 79) H.I., 72-year-old woman. Bowen's disease, area of onset, right auricle: *a,* preoperative condition; *b,* findings following tumor excision; *c,* condition following repair of the operation defect with the aid of a retroauricular skin flap; *d,* condition 4 months postoperatively.

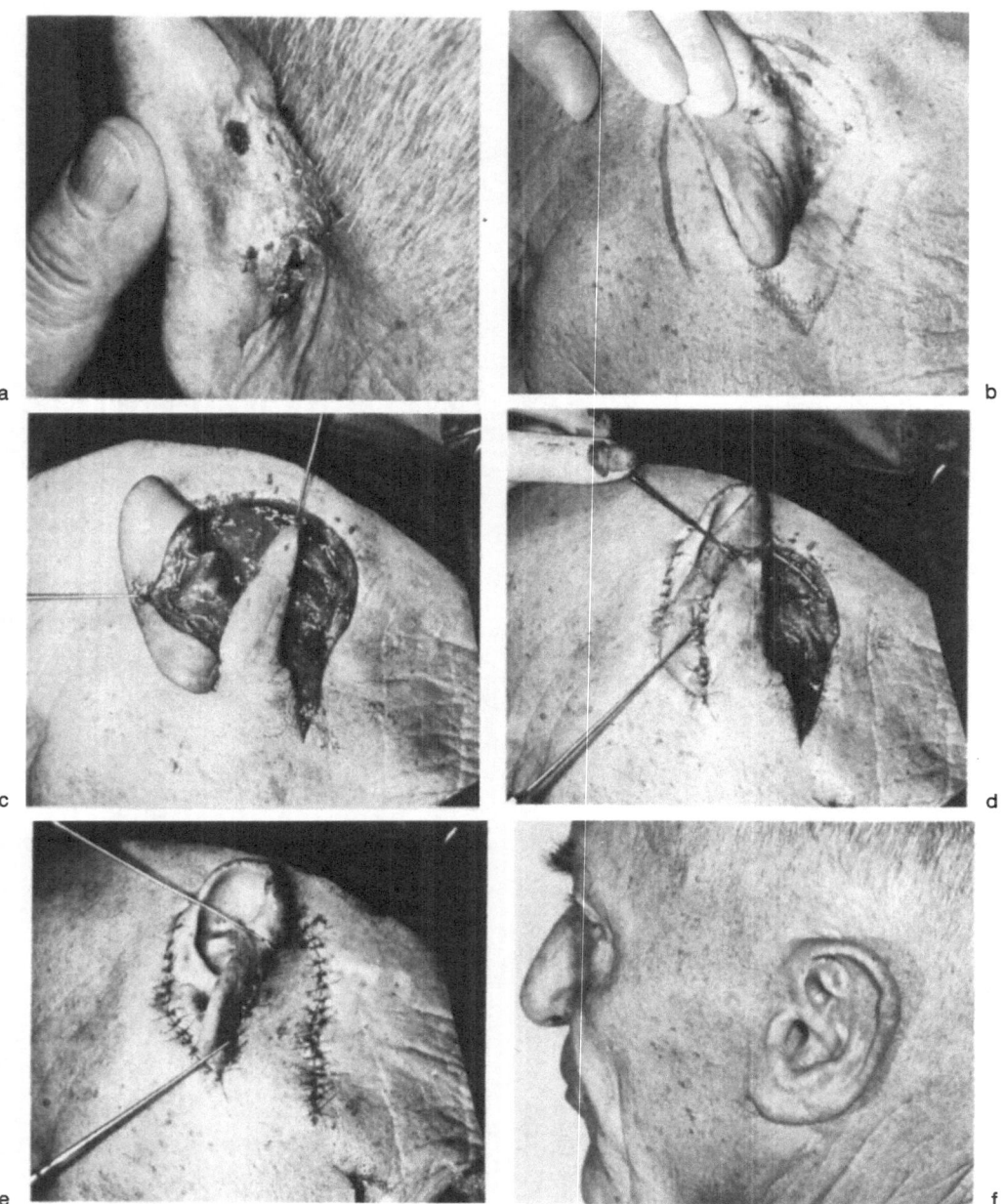

Plate 24. (cf. p. 79) H.F., 67-year-old man. Retroauricular basal cell carcinoma: *a,* preoperative condition; *b,* planning the operation—preauricular transposition flaps; *c,* transposition flaps placed in the operation defect after the partial resection of the conchal cartilage; *d,* condition after partial closure of the wound; *e,* condition at the end of the operation; *f,* condition 1 year postoperatively.

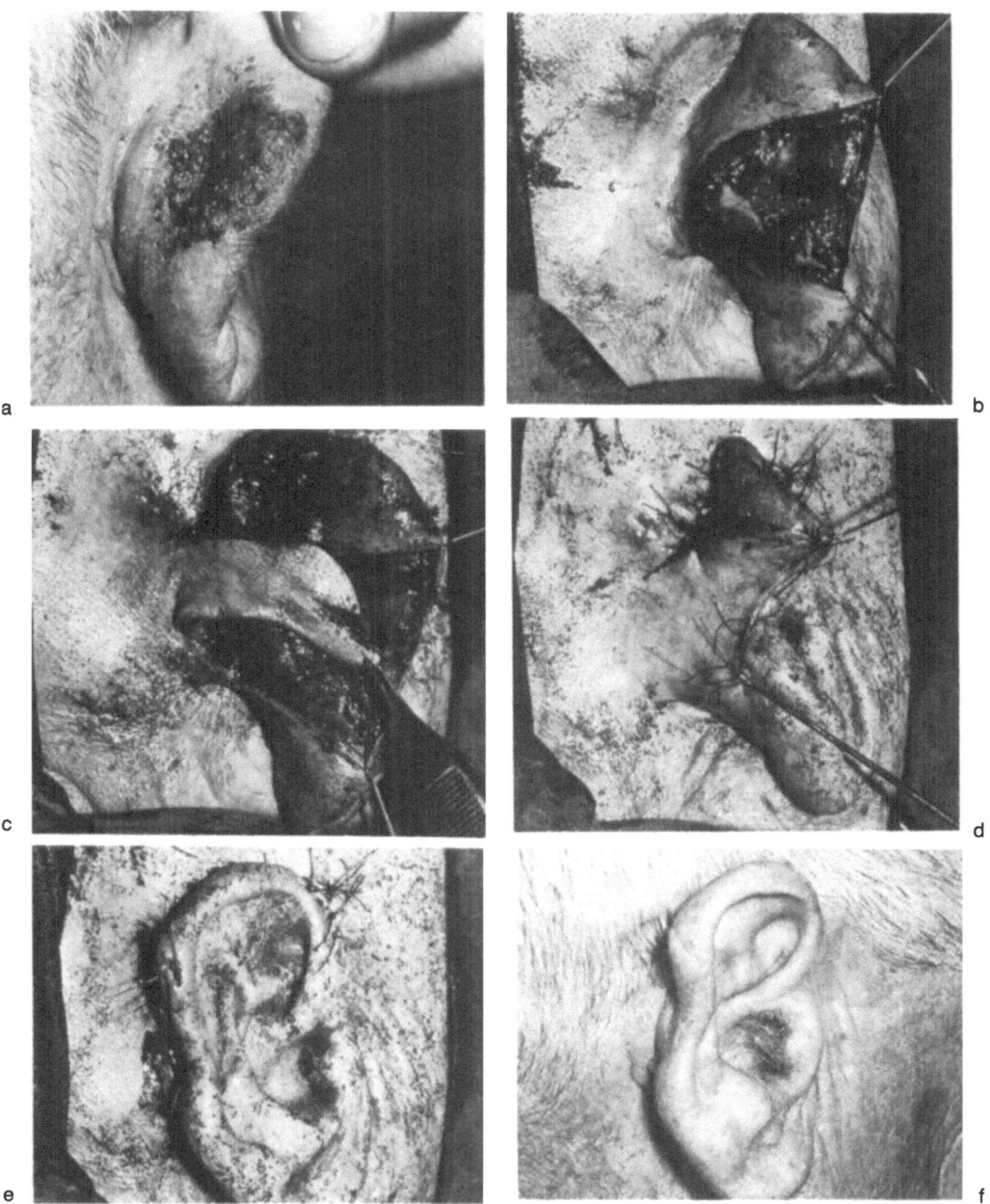

Plate 25. (cf. p. 79) G.H., 75-year-old man. Basal cell carcinoma of the back of the ear: *a*, preoperative condition; *b*, operation defect after the partial resection of the conchal cartilage; *c*, supraauricular transposition flaps placed in the operation defect; *d*, and *e*, condition at the end of the operation; *f*, condition 3 years postoperatively.

145

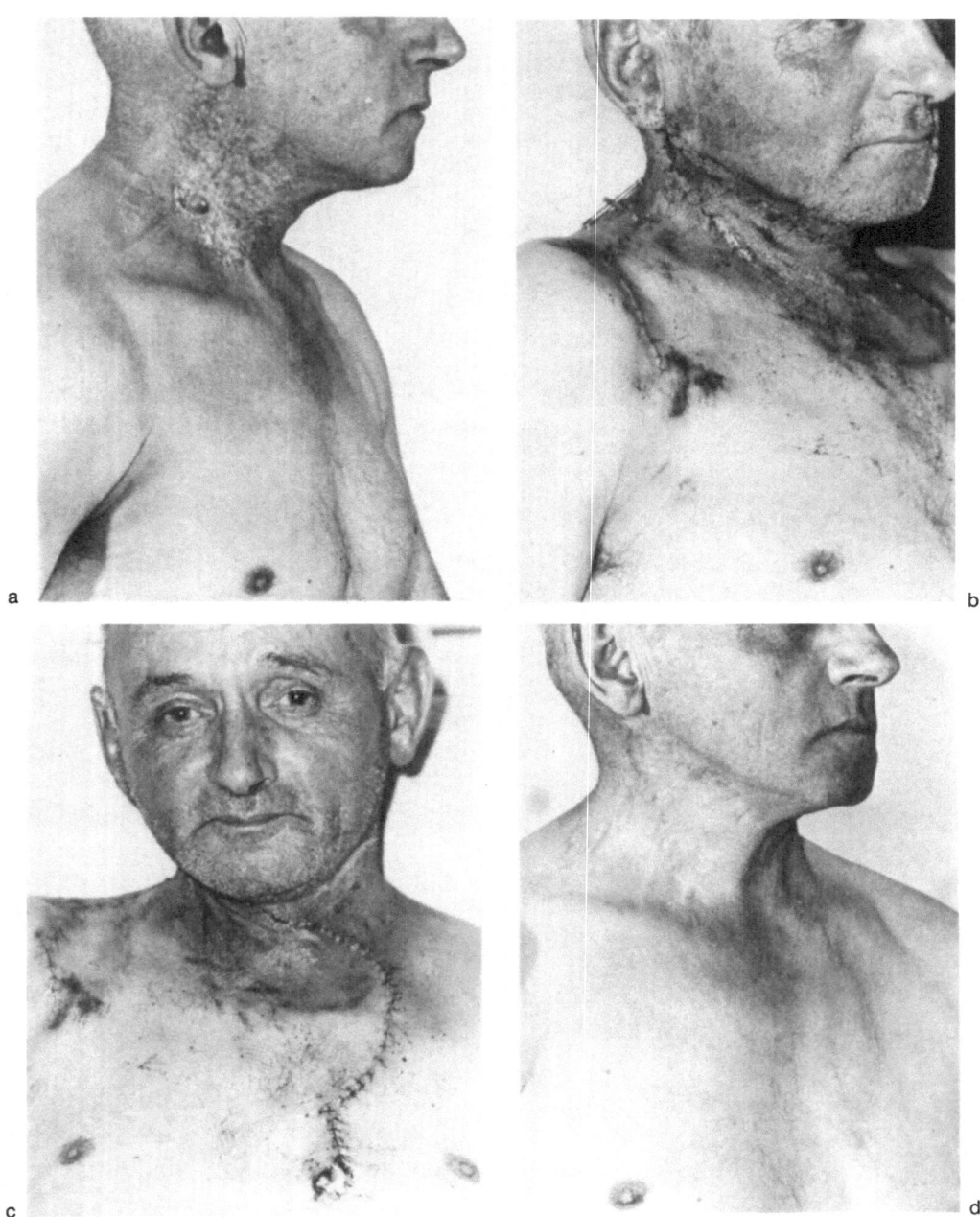

Plate 26. (cf. p. 82) M.F., 60-year-old man. Squamous cell carcinoma at the base of an old radiation scar on the right side of the neck. Radiation treatment had been performed 16 years before because of an actinic mycosis: *a,* preoperative condition; *b* and *c,* result 8 days after excision of the focus including the entire radiation field and defect repair by means of a double rotation flap from the shoulder and chest; *d,* condition 18 months postoperatively.

146

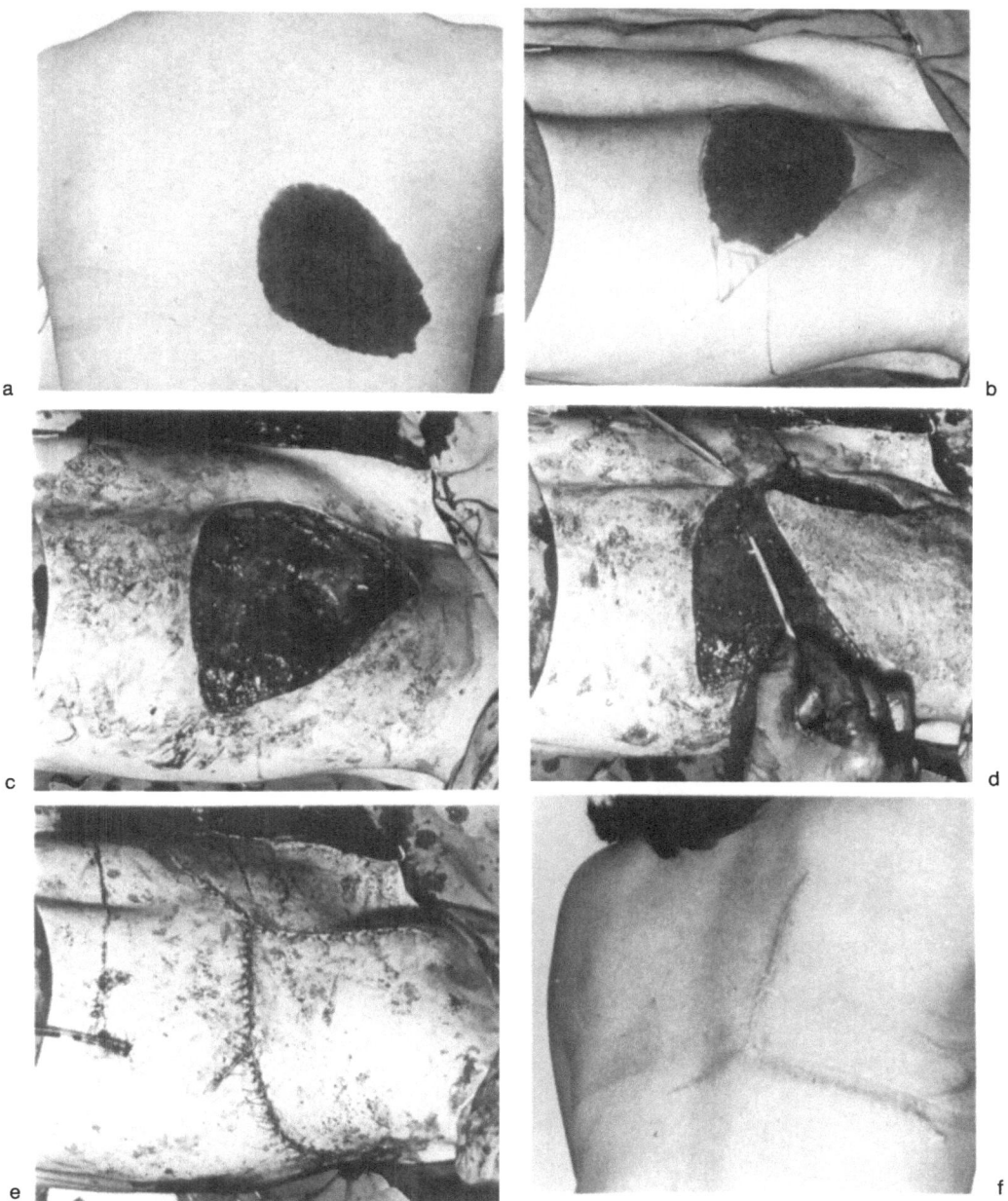

Plate 27. (cf. p. 83) 28-year-old woman. Hairy nevus in the area of the right half of the back: *a* and *b*, preoperative condition; *c*, after excision of the focus; *d*, rotation flap brought into the operation defect; *e*, operation defect closed by a rotation flap; *f*, condition 6 months postoperatively.

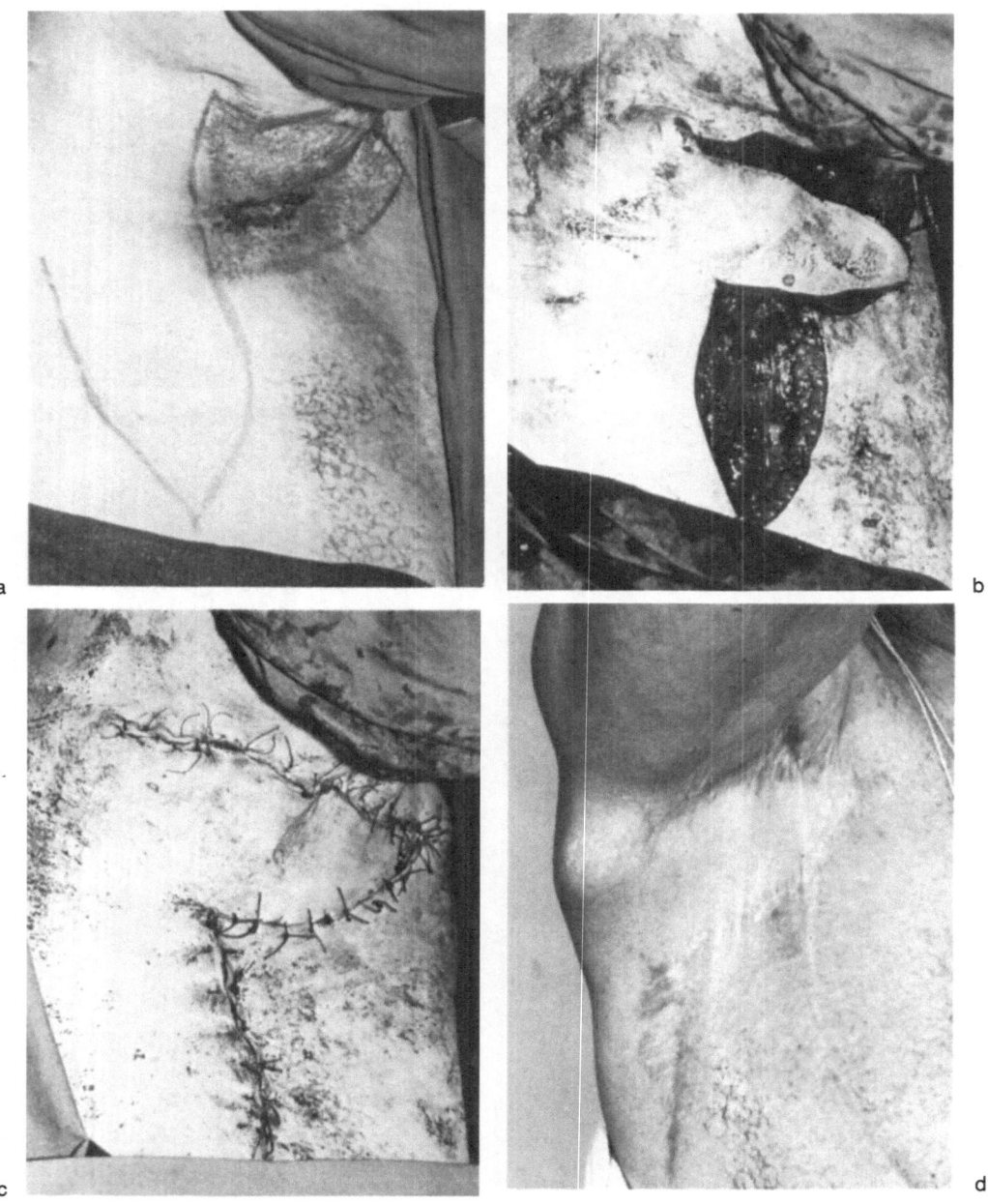

Plate 28. (cf. p. 83, 85) D.M., 73-year-old woman. Radiation ulcer of the right armpit: *a*, operation technique—transposition flaps from the lateral wall of the thorax; *b*, transposition flaps placed in the primary operation defect; *c*, condition at the end of the operation; *d*, condition 3 years postoperatively.

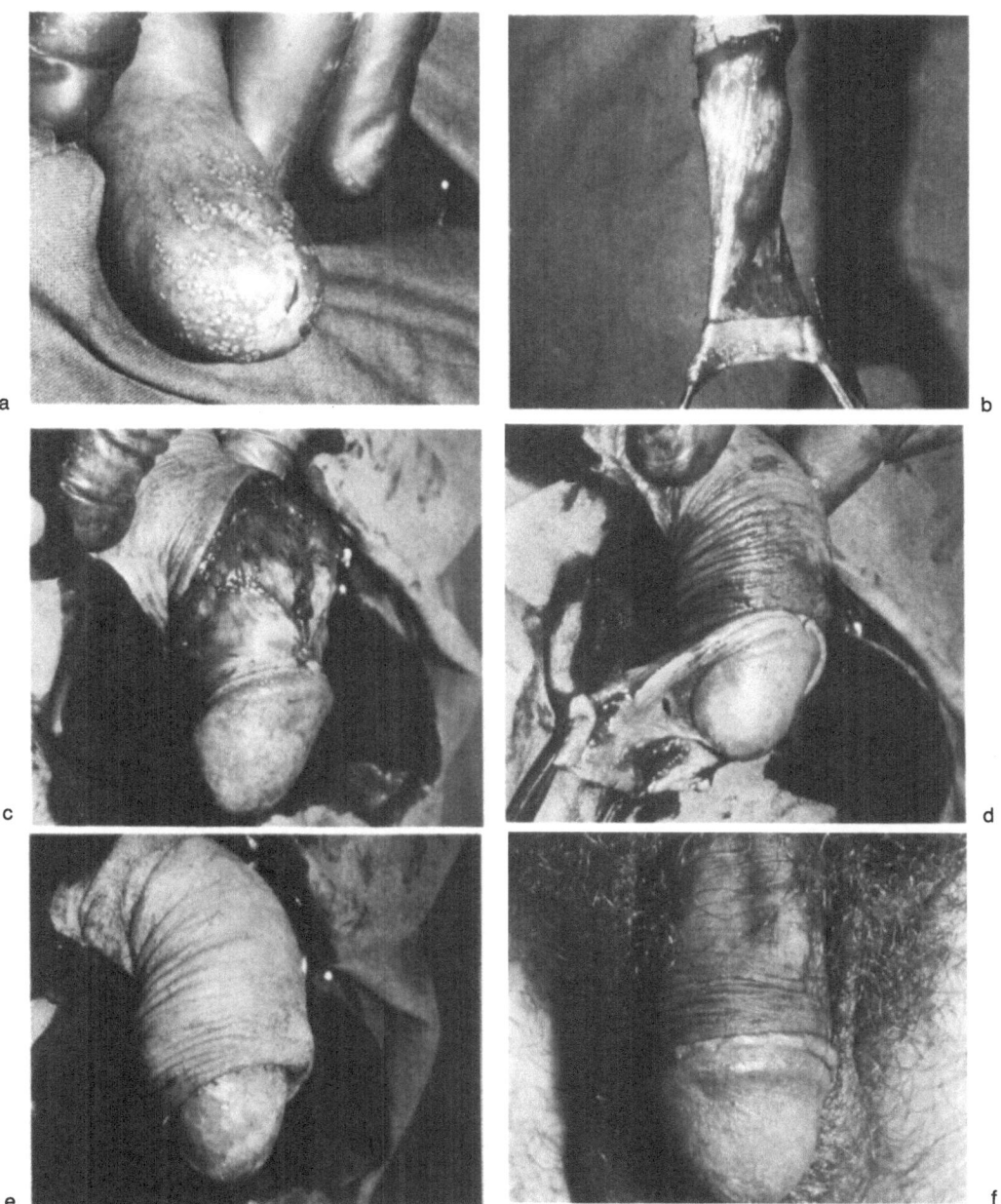

Plate 29. (cf. p. 87) S.U., 16-year-old boy. Phimosis: *a*, preoperative condition; *b*, using Rebreyoud's technique, condition after the separation of the outer from the inner foreskin; *c*, presentation of the inner foreskin; *d*, condition after resection of the inner foreskin in the vicinity of the sulcus; *e*, condition at the end of the operation; *f*, final condition 3 years postoperatively.

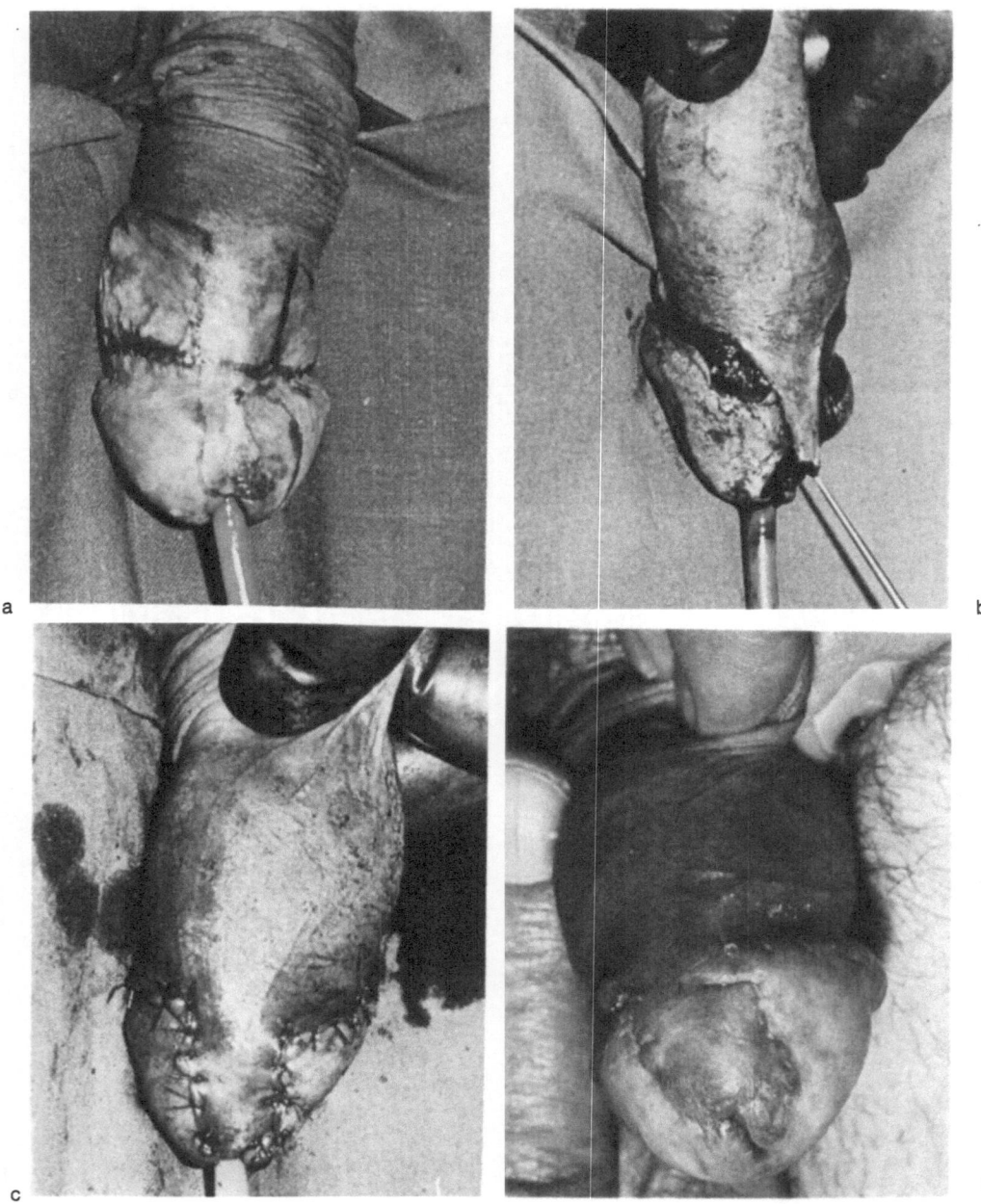

a

b

c

d

Plate 30. (cf. p. 88) A.L., 57-year-old man. Bowen's disease of the penis: *a*, condition before the skin flap operation using Happle's technique; *b*, condition after the excision of the tumor and the placing of the pedicled preputial flap in the primary operation defect; *c*, condition at the end of the operation; *d*, condition 6 weeks postoperatively.

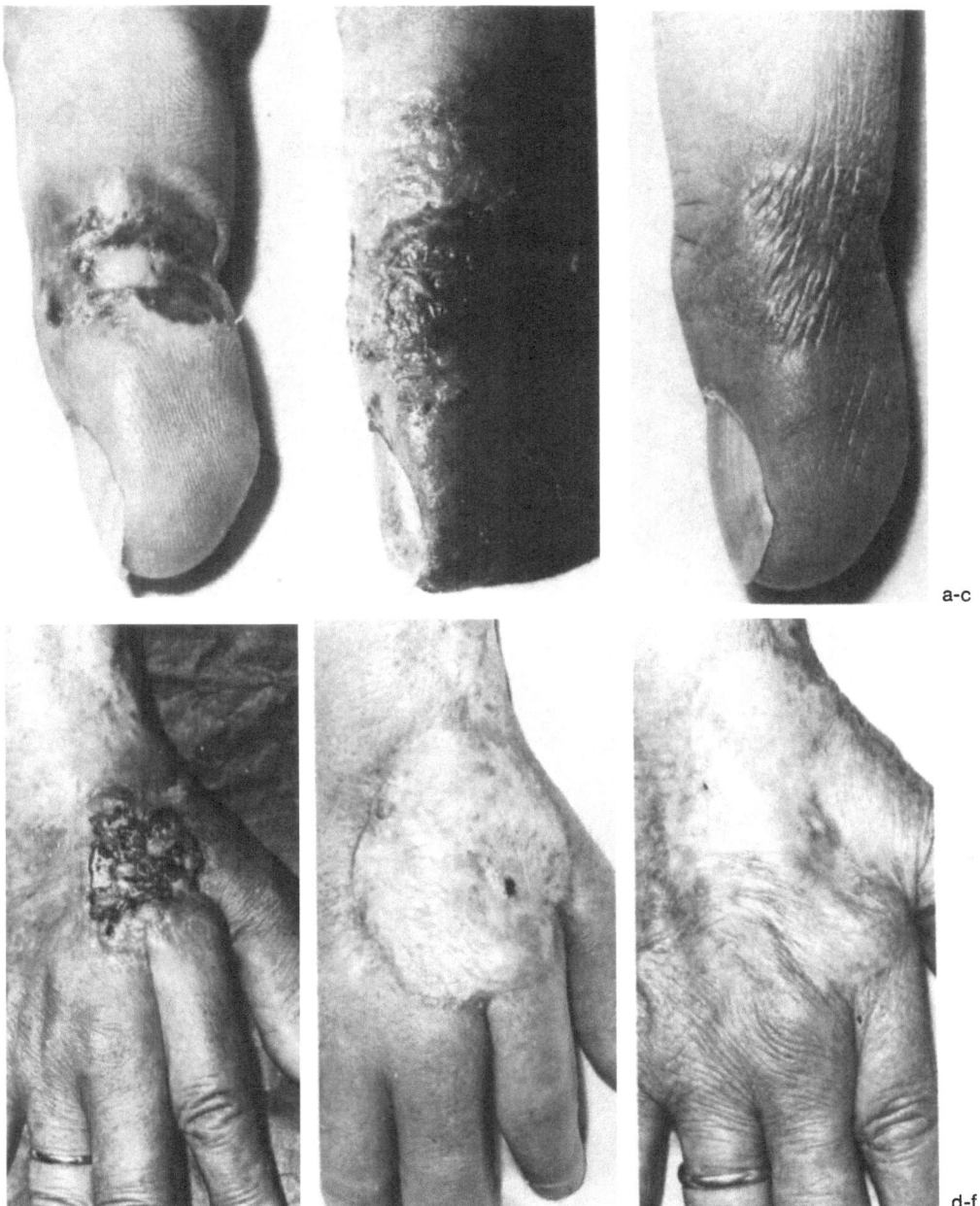

a-c

d-f

Plate 31. (cf. p. 92) (*a–c*) 50-year-old man. Radiation ulcer on the second left finger after radiation treatment for a wart 7 years before: *a*, preoperative condition; *b*, ten days after excision of the focus and repair of the defect with a free autologous full-thickness graft (livid coloration of the transplant); *c*, condition 2 years postoperatively.

(*d–f*) T.M., 66-year-old woman. Squamous cell carcinoma which had developed on the back of the left hand at the base of a scar following scalding during childhood: *d*, preoperative condition; *e*, two months postoperatively; *f*, condition 14 months postoperatively.

151

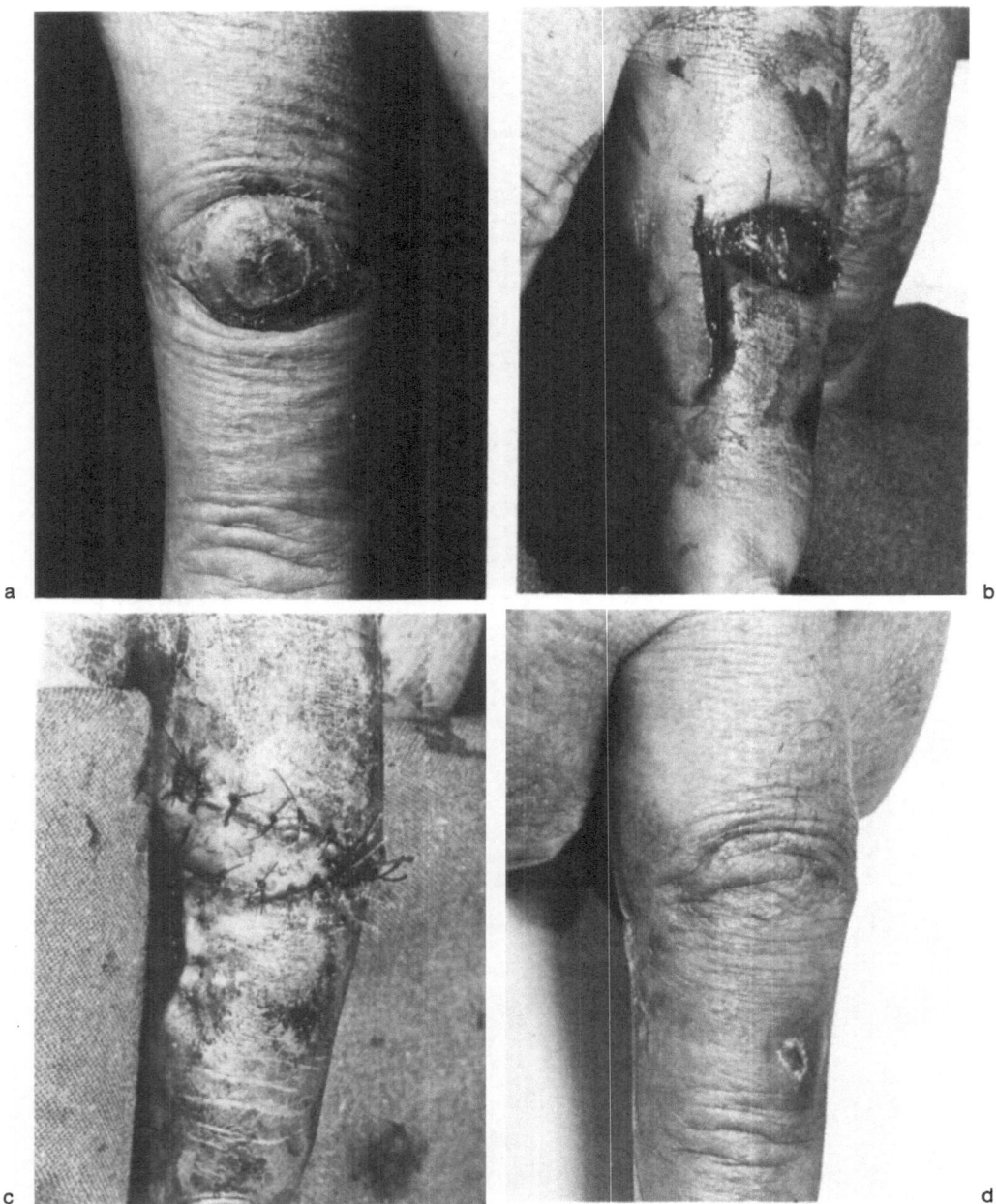

Plate 32. (cf. p. 92) H.W., 49-year-old man. Verruca vulgaris over the proximal interphalangeal joint of the fourth left finger, which had resisted therapy for several years: *a*, preoperative condition; *b*, after excision of the focus; *c*, findings following repair of the operation defect by means of a transposition flap from the medial side of the finger; flap donor site closed by primary sutures; *d*, result 10 months postoperatively.